W9-BYJ-117

STOP AMERICA'S #1 KILLER!

Reversible Vitamin Deficiency

Found to be Origin of

ALL Coronary Heart Disease

Thomas E. Levy, MD, JD

STOP AMERICA'S #1 KILLER!

Copyright © 2006 by Thomas E. Levy, M.D., J.D.

Library of Congress Control Number: 2006923883

ISBN: 0-9779520-0-2

All rights reserved. No part of this book may be reproduced or transmitted in any form or by any means, electronic or mechanical, including photocopying, recording, or by any information storage and retrieval system, without permission in writing from the copyright owner.

This book was printed in the United States of America.

To order additional copies of this book, contact:

Livon Books
1-800-334-9294
www.LivOnBooks.com
Orders@LivOnBooks.com
2654 W. Horizon Ridge Pkwy - Suite B-5, Dept 108
Henderson, NV 89052

To all those doctors — past, present, and future —
who dare to think for themselves.

ACKNOWLEDGMENTS

I would like to thank Les and Cindy Nachman of LivonLabs in Henderson, Nevada for their friendship and their gracious support of my work. Without their backing, this book may never have been completed and published. Any professional and/or commercial success that this book may eventually enjoy will need to be attributed to these two individuals.

Similarly, Dave Nicol of LivonLabs has not only been invaluable in backing my work along with Les and Cindy, he has helped immensely in putting the book and its concepts into a much more reader-friendly format for the benefit of all who obtain a copy. I think that I even understood my own work better after Dave had completed his revisions.

A thank you also goes to Shari Owenby of Livon-Labs for her able assistance with all of my interactions with LivonLabs.

Finally, I wish to offer a very special thanks to Dr. Julian Whitaker who wrote the Foreword to this book after reviewing it. Julian has been a friend and colleague for some years now, and having the support and positive feedback of such a distinguished physician and medical educator is extremely important and much appreciated.

FOREWORD

by Julian Whitaker, M.D.

In the mid-1960s, Nobel Laureate Linus Pauling began to study elements such as vitamin C, niacin, folic acid, and a number of other substances we now collectively call vitamins. It fascinated him that these elements could be used therapeutically in doses often a thousand times that found in food. In 1968, Pauling coined the term orthomolecular medicine and defined it as the use of elements common and essential to the body in various dosages to prevent and treat illness.

Whereas vitamin and mineral supplementation is common practice today, it is brand new to human history. That's because prior to the middle part of the 20th century there was no way to synthesize or extract vitamins and nutrients from other substances. In fact, the accurate molecular structure of vitamin C, one of the simpler vitamins, wasn't nailed down until the mid-30s. The discovery of these orthomolecular substances and their subsequent utilization in the prevention and treatment of disease is, in my opinion, the greatest medical advancement of the 20th century.

Unfortunately, the medical "business" is virtually owned by the pharmaceutical interests. Drug companies must patent the molecular structure of the active ingredient of their products in order to make a profit. Orthomolecular substances cannot be patented because they exist in nature. What does this mean? Nearly all prescription drugs, with the exception of some hormones, are not only substances not found in the human body — they are foreign to life!

Yet, these patented drugs enable the pharmaceutical companies to garner truly obscene profits. This money allows them to buy and spread influence in virtually every area of our society. Each year Big Pharma spends a whopping $16 billion on direct-to-physician promotion and another $4 billion peddling their wares directly to consumers through advertising. Consequently, the thought of utilizing orthomolecular substances to prevent and treat disease is not only forgotten but scorned by practitioners who are easy prey for the pharmaceutical industry.

The irony is that if an orthomolecular substance works today, it will work a million years from now. This cannot be said for the prescription drugs of today, many of which will be nonexistent only 100 years from now — if that long.

One barrier to physicians and individuals using orthomolecular substances is that they contradict the elements of style. That is to say, we all want and desire the latest and greatest. We look to new drugs with irrational hope. A "true breakthrough" hits the market, everyone rushes to try it, and when it fails yet another blockbuster drug takes its place. It's a vicious cycle. Orthomolecular substances, however, are found to have an increasing value rather than the decreasing value of drugs. In other words, vitamin C is not just for scurvy anymore.

The discovery of broadening benefits of orthomolecular substances is truly exciting, and Thomas Levy, MD, JD, is on the forefront in educating us on the positive effects of regular, large doses of one of the most remarkable orthomolecular substances: vitamin C.

In his first book on vitamin C, *Curing the Incurable*, Dr. Levy educated us on the use of vitamin C for the treatment of infections and toxins. This book opens our eyes to the almost unbelievable value this vitamin has in treating and preventing cardiovascular disease, our nation's deadliest killer.

Every aspect of the paradigm of elevated cholesterol being the culprit in cardiovascular disease, along with hypertension accelerating the process, is effectively dismantled by Dr. Levy's precise information on the role vitamin C plays in all heart risk factors. The mechanism of atherosclerosis, outlined by Dr. Levy, showing that the absence of vitamin C causes connective tissue of the wall of the arteries to become mushy and watery allowing penetration of foreign substances, is both intriguing and convincing.

In his last chapter he points out convincing evidence from a recent study which demonstrates that slightly increasing your vitamin C tissue concentration reduces all causes of mortality. This decrease is continuous and inversely proportional to the level of vitamin C maintained in the system. People with the highest vitamin C levels had the lowest death rate from all causes, and this reduction in death rate was independent of the presence or absence of other risk factors.

Dr. Levy should be commended and applauded. He has put an enormous amount of effort into convincing us of the benefits of ingesting high volumes of vitamin C, which constitutes virtually no effort. It is amazing that a practice of such simplicity, such ease, and such little negative consequence could have such a magnitude of benefits in combating our more serious and deadly diseases. The message of Dr. Levy's book is very simple: Substantially increase your levels of vitamin C, keep them up to par, and live well and long.

TABLE OF CONTENTS

Section One

How to Stop America's #1 Killer: Attacking Causes, Not Symptoms

CHAPTER 1

It's Time for a Unifying Perspective of Heart Disease

*The art of healing comes from nature and not from
the physician. Therefore, the physician must
start from nature with an open mind.*

PARACELSUS

Today, heart disease, primarily coronary heart disease, remains unchallenged as the leading cause of death throughout the world. This book will scientifically demonstrate that atherosclerosis — the buildup of plaque in the arteries which leads to heart attacks — is easily preventable and even reversible.

Furthermore, this book will also demonstrate that heart disease, one of the most complex and frequently researched topics in all of medicine, is not so difficult to understand when looked at from a different, unifying perspective.

Simply stated, atherosclerosis is a disease that appears to be initiated by a deficiency of vitamin C in the innermost lining of the arteries. This innermost lining, called the intima, once damaged by a lack of vitamin C, initiates and stimulates a host of different plaque-building processes. The mechanisms that are set in motion for any particular individual depend on a variety of different cardiac risk factors, but the result, arterial blockage, is always the same.

Scurvy, the disease that results from insufficient vitamin C intake over an extended period of time, is usually thought of as a condition that affects the entire body equally. Clinically, scurvy is characterized by weakness, anemia, and a tendency to have easy bleeding into the tissues, especially the gums. In fact, scurvy is very often a much more localized, focal process. While focal scurvy does typically require some degree of generalized vitamin C deficiency in the body, the overall body can clinically appear very healthy with specific areas of the body nevertheless severely deficient in vitamin C.

An individual with advanced periodontal disease, an example of a focal scurvy as determined by gum biopsy specimens, will not usually display the classical symptoms of scurvy in the rest of the body. Another localized disease, cataracts, can be considered a form of focal scurvy in the cornea. Similarly, atherosclerosis can readily be characterized as "arterial scurvy," because the lack of vitamin C in the arterial linings appears to always be the first identifiable starting point for the development of coronary heart disease.

How does a focal scurvy occur in the midst of what would normally be considered sufficient vitamin C intake? The fact is, there are known conditions in the body that can accelerate the depletion of vitamin C in certain tissues and structures. This is certainly the case in arterial scurvy.

For this reason, the treatment of arterial scurvy, while straightforward, requires attention to details other than simple vitamin C supplementation. For many different reasons, regular vitamin C supplementation is of benefit to nearly everyone, and the general health can be expected to improve even if no other interventions are taken. However, it is important to understand why a given person has low levels of vitamin C in their arterial linings in the first place.

In almost every case, the cause of low vitamin C levels in the arterial linings is a significant daily toxin exposure. These toxins keep neutralizing (oxidizing) the body's stores of vitamin C making the maintenance of active (reduced or non-oxidized) vitamin C levels in the various tissues of the body virtually impossible.

The arterial intima is especially prone to this localized deficiency. Whenever any toxins are released into the blood, the inner lining of the arteries is logically one of the first "destinations" for the toxins to gather and start neutralizing local vitamin C stores, at least partly explaining why arterial scurvy is probably the most common form of focal scurvy.

This is why the practical suggestions portion of this book might initially seem so overly involved or detailed. The proper removal of dental toxicity, especially root canal-treated teeth, is absolutely essential for minimizing an otherwise very large source of daily toxicity. Nutrition to minimize daily toxin exposure absorbed from the gut is also extremely important. When the lion's share of daily toxin exposure to the body has been brought to a reasonable minimum, quality supplementation is freed of its burden to neutralize a large and relentless toxin exposure. Then, and only then, can the natural healing of the blood vessel proceed as the antioxidant and nutrient status of its inner wall becomes optimized.

So, prepare to be amazed, especially if you are a health care practitioner who has always felt that atherosclerosis is largely an unstoppable and steadily progressive disease. It is not. An objective review of the available scientific evidence demonstrates otherwise. Turn an abnormal coronary angiogram into a normal one. What is now considered a rare but theoretically possible occurrence can now become an expected outcome.

CHAPTER 2
The Genesis of Arterial Narrowings and Blockages

In order to fully appreciate why arterial narrowings develop, you must have a reasonable understanding of the anatomy of a normal blood vessel. You will also need to know what it takes to produce and maintain a normal blood vessel. You may be tempted to pass over this "technical" information, but it will be of immeasurable benefit if you take the time to comprehend what is presented here.

THE NORMAL ARTERY

The discussion here will be restricted to the largest arteries in the body and the smallest ones, the capillaries. Both of these types of blood vessels are the most significant players in the development of atherosclerosis. It is also important to realize that the arteries of the body are the blood vessels that deliver the blood away from the heart. The blood pressure required to pump your blood into the tissues farthest from the heart exerts great stress on all the vessels on the arterial side of circulation with the greatest pressure occurring in the largest arteries close to the heart.

These arterial vessels gradually decrease in diameter until they become capillaries. Capillaries are so small that blood cells can only pass through in single file. As the blood continues to travel through the capillaries, the vessels gradually increase in size becoming the veins on the venous half of the body's circulation. It is the venous system that returns blood to the heart and lungs for reoxygenation and redistribution throughout the body via the arterial system.

EXHIBIT 1

The vessels exposed to the highest blood pressure, the arteries, are the most prone to atherosclerosis.

The venous system requires much less blood pressure to move your blood back to the heart than is found in the arterial system. The much higher blood pressure in the arterial system is likely one of the primary reasons that arteries are far more prone to develop thickenings of the vessel walls with subsequent narrowings or blockages. In fact, the largest arteries develop most of the atherosclerosis, and the largest arteries are the blood vessels that must deal with the highest of blood pressures.

As the arteries get smaller and eventually taper down to the capillary level, the blood pressure in those vessels also gets progressively lower. The smaller arteries get much less atherosclerosis, and the disease is rarely seen at the capillary level. High blood pressure, then, appears to be directly associated with atherosclerosis, and it is probably one of the primary factors in its development.

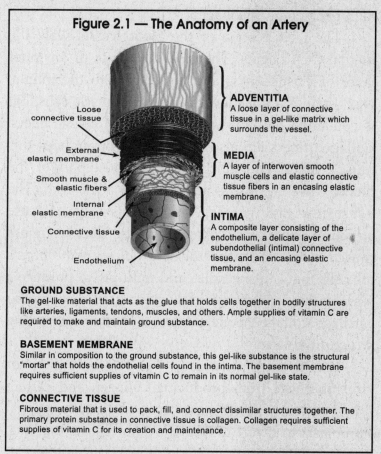

Figure 2.1 — The Anatomy of an Artery

Loose connective tissue

External elastic membrane

Smooth muscle & elastic fibers

Internal elastic membrane

Connective tissue

Endothelium

ADVENTITIA
A loose layer of connective tissue in a gel-like matrix which surrounds the vessel.

MEDIA
A layer of interwoven smooth muscle cells and elastic connective tissue fibers in an encasing elastic membrane.

INTIMA
A composite layer consisting of the endothelium, a delicate layer of subendothelial (intimal) connective tissue, and an encasing elastic membrane.

GROUND SUBSTANCE
The gel-like material that acts as the glue that holds cells together in bodily structures like arteries, ligaments, tendons, muscles, and others. Ample supplies of vitamin C are required to make and maintain ground substance.

BASEMENT MEMBRANE
Similar in composition to the ground substance, this gel-like substance is the structural "mortar" that holds the endothelial cells found in the intima. The basement membrane requires sufficient supplies of vitamin C to remain in its normal gel-like state.

CONNECTIVE TISSUE
Fibrous material that is used to pack, fill, and connect dissimilar structures together. The primary protein substance in connective tissue is collagen. Collagen requires sufficient supplies of vitamin C for its creation and maintenance.

The anatomy of the normal artery is fairly straightforward (Ross, 1992). The thickness of the arterial wall is composed of three basic layers: the intima, the media, and the adventitia. The *intima* is the innermost layer directly surrounding the blood flow, and it is composed primarily of a thin layer of connective tissue with a coating layer of cells (endothelium) that directly contacts your blood. This thin connective tissue layer consists primarily of what is known as basement membrane, which contains a high percentage of collagen.

The next portion of the blood vessel wall, the media, then begins. The *media* consists of an inner layer of elastic fibers and is adjacent to the intima. Next there is a thick layer of smooth muscle cells that is contained by another, outer layer of elastic fibers. Collagen fibers are also interspersed throughout this muscle layer. The third and outermost part of the blood vessel wall, the adventitia, is then seen. The *adventitia* (add-ven-TEE-sha) consists of a dense structure containing collagen, elastic fibers, smooth muscle cells, and numerous fibroblasts. *Fibroblasts* are cells that can specialize and multiply to produce a wide variety of different connective tissues, including cartilage, collagen, bone, tendon, and other supporting structural tissues.

A vitamin C deficiency will not only slow or stop fibroblsts from producing collagen and certain other proteins, it will also cause mature, functional fibroblasts to revert to immature fibroblasts that lack tissue-specific functions (Gould, 1963). This effect of vitamin C deficiency may play a very important role in the origin of several types of cancer.

The cells which comprise the blood vessels are surrounded by an intercellular glue known as ground substance. *Ground substance* is the mortar that holds many of your body's tissues together. It has essentially the same composition as the basement membrane and it serves as a gel-like framework into which connective tissue cells and fibers are embedded. The ground substance contains a large quantity of very large molecules known as glycoproteins. *Glycoproteins* are composed of a protein and a carbohydrate that, in the presence of vitamin C, interconnect to form a thick gel (polymerization) that acts as the "glue" that binds most of the cells in the body together.

> **EXHIBIT 2**
> Vitamin C is essential for producing and maintaining the intercellular glue that keeps arteries strong and intact.

The concept that the ground substance has such a gel-like consistency was held by multiple earlier investigators (Clark and Clark, 1918 and 1933; Laguesse, 1921; Bensley, 1934; McMasters and Parsons, 1939).

Vitamin C is essential to maintain the strength of this intercellular glue (Pauling, 1983). The interconnected, gel-like nature of the molecules in the intercellular cement tends to be optimal when vitamin C levels are optimal. When vitamin C is deficient, the interconnections are broken (depolymerization), and the intercellular glue, in ground substance and basement membranes, loses its gel-like nature and becomes loose, runny, and watery.

This loss of the gel-like consistency of the ground substance in the face of vitamin C deficiency was reported by Wolbach and Howe (1926). Kefalides (1968) also noted that the basement membrane in blood vessels appeared to contain a protein either very similar or identical to the collagen of bone and connective tissue.

Priest (1970), looking at mouse cells in culture, found that vitamin C stimulated the formation of the basement membrane, while scurvy conditions restricted its formation.

Berenson (1961) put it another way, noting "that the normal biochemistry of units which compose connective tissue is of major importance in maintenance of the integrity of the cardiovascular system."

EXHIBIT 3

Vitamin C deficiency has been shown to breakdown the "intercellular glue" into components that "leak" into the blood.

Gersh and Catchpole (1949) suggested that the level of glycoproteins in the blood was a direct reflection of the state, or health, of the intercellular glue surrounding the tissues of the body. Higher blood glycoprotein levels were considered reflective of a poorer status, or greater abnormality.

A bit later, Pirani and Catchpole (1951) proposed that the "ungelled" molecules (depolymerized or fragmented glycoproteins) from the intercellular glue readily gained access to the blood when their interconnections were dissolved due to vitamin C deficiency. They showed that guinea pigs with either acute or chronic scurvy had elevated levels of these molecules in the blood. Furthermore, they demonstrated that the administration of vitamin C decreased their levels in the blood. This directly implies that the integrity of the intercellular glue (ground substance) had been

EXHIBIT 4

Administration of vitamin C has been shown to decrease the "leakage" of "intercellular glue" components into the blood.

restored by the vitamin C and the smaller, previously disconnected glycoproteins were no longer "leaking" into the blood.

Fisher et al. (1991) found that vitamin C is needed for the production of both glycoproteins* and collagen by fibroblasts. This relatively recent study helps to confirm the validity of the much earlier work by Wolbach and Howe (1926), Gersh and Catchpole (1949), and Pirani and Catchpole (1951) indicating that vitamin C is essential for maintaining the integrity of the glycoprotein-containing ground substance.

EXHIBIT 5

When the intercellular glue in the arteries becomes watery due to the lack of vitamin C, the first step of atherosclerosis has taken place.

When the intercellular glue in your arteries becomes watery due to the lack of vitamin C, the first step of atherosclerosis has taken place.

Early on, when little further change has taken place, the process can be completely reversed in a very short period of time with the proper replenishment of vitamin C. When the atherosclerotic process has evolved further, it is still reversible, although the degree of reversal tends to lessen and the amount of time to achieve that reversal tends to be greater.

EXHIBIT 6

All three layers in arterial walls require the normal formation of collagen to remain healthy and strong.

Another important point to take away from this brief anatomy lesson on the arterial wall is that all

---

*The terminology for glycoprotein is not consistent in the literature. In this case, the researchers often appeared to use the term proteoglycan as a synonym for glycoprotein.

three layers in the wall require the normal formation and maintenance of collagen in order to be an anatomically normal structure. Buddecke (1962) noted that the "arterial wall corresponds in its morphological structure to a formed connective tissue."

Vitamin C is absolutely essential for the normal formation of collagen throughout your body (Gould, 1958; Ohlwiler et al., 1960; Barnes, 1969). Furthermore, adequate amounts of vitamin C are essential for the proper maintenance of normal collagen previously created in the presence of adequate vitamin C. All cells and tissues in the body undergo some degree of turnover and metabolism, requiring an ongoing supply of nutrients, especially vitamin C.

EXHIBIT 7

Vitamin C is required for the normal production and maintenance of collagen throughout the body.

Collagens are the most abundant proteins in the human body, constituting about 30% of the body's total protein content. Probably the single most important characteristic of collagen is that it physically has a stiff, strong nature. This characteristic literally allows collagen to give the tissues in which it is predominant a substantial mechanical strength, resistant to rupture or significant distortion.

Tissues containing significant amounts of collagen include tendons, ligaments, cornea, lens, skin, bone, teeth, cartilage, heart valves, blood vessels, smooth muscles, basement membranes, gut, and some organs. Collagen is also an important constituent in many of the tissue spaces surrounding cells (the extracellular framework, also occupied by the ground substance), where it is not organized into any of the defined tissue types noted in the previous paragraph.

Another aspect of the arterial system that is involved in the later stages of atherosclerotic blockages is the capillary system. Capillaries develop inside advanced atherosclerotic blockages of significant bulk so that the blockages can have some blood supply of their own and not die (become necrotic). However, this will often result in the exposure of capillaries to blood pressure levels not normally encountered by the capillary system. This exposure of the structurally frail capillaries to unusually high blood pressure can result in the rupture of these small blood vessels. When the capillaries are present in an advanced, bulky atherosclerotic plaque, their rupture can result in bleeding into the plaque itself, sometimes resulting in a sudden, total blockage of the artery as that area quickly expands (Paterson, 1936, 1938, and 1941).

Structurally, the capillary is like a blood vessel composed of intima only, much like the internal lining of a large artery without the other two supporting layers. Furthermore, the diameter of the capillary is very tiny, often requiring single red blood cells to bend a bit in order to pass through. Essentially, as the larger arteries taper down to the capillary level, only the intima layer is retained, since capillaries are not normally expected to withstand the high blood pressures found in the arteries close to the heart.

WHY ARTERIAL NARROWINGS DEVELOP

Arterial narrowing refers to a decrease in the internal diameter (caliber) of the blood vessel. When the narrowing gets restrictive enough, the blood flow downstream from the narrowing is decreased. Narrowing results as the wall surrounding the blood vessel thickens,* thus reducing the size of the internal passageway.

A number of different factors can play a role in whether an arterial narrowing develops. Practically all of the seemingly diverse factors causing atherosclerotic wall thickenings in the arteries end up inflicting their effects either directly or indirectly through the consequences of vitamin C deficiency. In a real sense, then, vitamin C deficiency appears to be the "final common pathway" that determines whether a given factor will cause an arterial narrowing to develop.

DEGENERATION: 1ST STAGE OF ATHEROSCLEROSIS

Probably the first significant change that takes place in the blood vessel wall in the face of a significant vitamin C deficiency is the ungelling of the glycoproteins in the basement membrane and the ground substance. Associated with this change, electron microscopy has revealed that the endothelial cells in scurvy-stricken guinea pigs begin to separate (Gore et al., 1965).

This "ungelling" of the "internal glue" can be considered the "degenerative" phase of atheroscle-

---

*There are several synonyms for this process of arterial thickening, including "lesion," "plaque," or "blockage."

rosis. This degeneration results in the leakage of the unlinked glycoproteins into the blood, and the gel-like consistency of the ground substance becomes loose and watery. As the ground substance loses its grip on the cells that line the interior wall, the blood vessel wall is "broken down," and the body then compensates by "thickening" the arterial wall.

Figure 2.2 — Early Progression of Arterial Scurvy

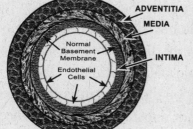

**ARTERIAL CROSS SECTION
NORMAL STATE**

Endothelial cells are firmly embedded in healthy, gelled basement membrane. Vitamin C is essential for the maintenance of the collagen and glycoproteins, as well as the normal "jelly-like" consistency of healthy basement membrane.

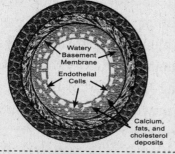

**ARTERIAL CROSS SECTION
"DEGENERATIVE STAGE"**

A deficiency of vitamin C changes the consistency of the basement membrane from "jelly-like" to watery. Substances normally in the blood, such as calcium, fats, and cholesterol are now able to more easily pass between the endothelial cells into the basement membrane. This causes a thickening of the intima and consequently a smaller arterial diameter.

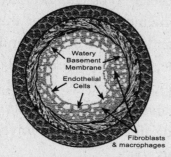

**ARTERIAL CROSS SECTION
"PROLIFERATIVE STAGE"**

In order to fortify the weakened arterial wall against eventual failure/rupture, the body activates fibroblasts (cells that generate collagen and fibers). At the same time, macrophages (a special type of white blood cell) enter the intima to "eat up" the invading deposits of cholesterol, calcium, and fats, All of this activity contributes to the noticeable thickening of the arterial wall.

It is felt that this breakdown of ground substance directly leads to a number of subsequent consequences. Gersh and Catchpole (1949) proposed that this change in the physical consistency of the ground substance must have an influence on the diffusion of both nutrients and metabolites between the cells of the blood vessels. They asserted that the normal, gel-like state of the ground substance tends to be water-insoluble, while the abnormal, ungelled state of the ground substance is very water-soluble. Such a change in the basic state of solubility can have very wide-ranging effects on what can and cannot diffuse into these areas.

Gersh and Catchpole also postulated that it is likely that the ungelling of the large interconnected molecules in the ground substance also produces smaller molecules. These smaller molecules have a greater chance of bonding to and/or interacting with the nutrients and waste products that normally pass between the cells and the blood in abnormal ways. Such interactions could dramatically hinder the ability of the endothelial cells lining the inside of the artery to block the penetration of unwanted substances and their subsequent deposition.

Recall that the endothelial cells are actually embedded in the basement membrane. Whether the basement membrane is firm and jelly-like or loose and watery will determine whether certain unwanted substances (like calcium, cholesterol, and fats) abnormally diffuse into the vessel wall, causing progressive thickening. As the initial stages of atherosclerosis evolve, such a thickening is commonly seen.

On the other hand, any factor that increases the thickness of the basement membrane (like calcium, cholesterol, and fats) can be expected to decrease the ability of beneficial substances dissolved in the blood (like vitamin C and other nutrients) to normally penetrate the vessel wall and reach deep into the tissues.

Gersh and Catchpole also suggested that this initial breakdown of the ground substance or basement membrane directly promotes the abnormal formation of calcium deposits within these substances. Even though hard, rock-like areas of calcification are not seen grossly until the latest stages of atherosclerosis, it is interesting to note that the predisposition to calcification with actual calcium deposition appears to begin very early in this disease.

PROLIFERATION: 2ND STAGE OF ATHEROSCLEROSIS

After the basement membrane/intercellular ground substance has lost its gel-like consistency and acquired new properties of increased water solubility, the next changes seen in the regular evolution of atherosclerosis can now take place. All of these subsequent changes of atherosclerosis can be lumped into what is known as the "proliferative" phase of atherosclerosis, which follows the initial "degenerative" changes noted above.

Soon after the ground substance ungels and lipids get deposited into it, an abundance of cells in the intimal area of the blood vessel will be seen to accumulate or proliferate. Typically these cells are macrophages, which are special white blood cells that serve to engulf, or "eat up," what the body interprets to be undesirable foreign bodies. In this case, the foreign bodies are the lipid deposits in the ground substance and basement membrane. As noted in the section on inflammation in Chapter 4, this influx of macrophages could also be a compensatory mechanism by the body to attempt to deliver vitamin C to areas of the blood vessel wall depleted of it. As more lipid gets deposited and more macrophages show up to ingest that lipid, the blood vessel wall begins to show a clear thickening at the sites that had initially been most depleted of vitamin C. This thickening of the intimal lining of the blood vessel is generally the first easily detectable indicator that atherosclerosis has begun to evolve.

What appears next in the evolution of atherosclerosis depends upon the immediate microenvironment surrounding the damaged basement membrane and ground substance. The presence of high circulating levels of cholesterol and lipoprotein(a) will produce one effect, while normal or even low circulating levels of these substances will produce another effect. Also, the presence of toxins and microbes in the blood will have its own effect on what happens next.

With the absence or significantly lessened presence of infectious agents and circulating toxins in the blood (e.g., from root canal-treated teeth or periodontal disease), the component of inflammation in the evolution of atherosclerosis can be expected to be much less pronounced. Although the very state of vitamin C deficiency likely helps to sustain the presence of inflammation in the atherosclerotic blood vessel wall (see

Chapter 4), the presence of infection and toxicity would be expected to make the inflammation risk factor for the development of atherosclerosis much more pronounced.

Infection and toxicity will also accelerate the rate at which vitamin C is depleted from the body (Levy, 2002) and the blood vessel wall.

Diphtheria toxin, which will substantially increase the rate of vitamin C depletion, seems to favor the development of a type of arteriosclerosis that focuses on the media (middle layer) of the artery in both the vitamin C-deprived guinea pig (Menten and King, 1935) and the normal guinea pig (Bailey, 1917). Menten and King also found that other infectious and infectious/toxic agents could produce thickening only in the arterial media while leaving the intima largely unaffected.

Interestingly, these investigators also found that the vitamin C-depleting diphtheria toxin produced a degeneration of the insulin-producing cells of the pancreas in the guinea pigs. This resulted in higher blood glucose levels. As will be repeatedly shown in this book, few risk factors operate completely independently, and toxins can clearly play a role as well in producing diabetes or aggravating pre-existing diabetes, which is a significant risk factor for atherosclerosis by itself.

The clinical picture resulting from any toxin will basically depend upon where the toxin biochemically is prone to accumulate, with the resulting vitamin C deficiency developing in that area of accumulation.

Finally, the degree of vitamin C deficiency will also be a significant factor determining the relative impact of other risk factors present at the time. Risk factors are not static processes; multiple factors can increase or even amplify the impact of each other, and this variability, combined with a greater or lesser deficiency of vitamin C, can produce differing evolutions of atherosclerosis. King and Menten (1935) reached a similar conclusion, noting that there is a "wide zone of vitamin C deficiency" short of scurvy, and that bacterial toxins such as diphtheria toxin can have variable levels of harmful effect depending upon the degree of vitamin C deficiency.

> **EXHIBIT 8**
>
> **The clinical picture resulting from any toxin is dependent upon where the toxin is prone to accumulate, with a focal vitamin C deficiency developing there.**

Lipids (e.g., cholesterol and lipoprotein(a)) begin to be deposited in the ground substance after the ungelling of the glycoproteins due to vitamin C deficiency has taken place. This lipid can initially be detected with the use of special staining for visualization with the microscope (Moon and Rinehart, 1952). The change in the physical restraint offered by a gel versus the physical restraint offered by a thin, watery substance appears to play a substantial role in allowing the uptake of the lipids circulating in the blood into the altered ground substance. Also, as noted earlier, the solubility characteristics of the basement membrane/ground substance change dramatically in the face of vitamin C deficiency, which directly affects whether the substances taken up from the blood remain in solution after getting into the basement membrane/ground substance area.

Overall, then, a focal vitamin C deficiency in the arterial wall "degenerates" the basement membrane allowing the abnormal deposition of solutes such as calcium, cholesterol, and fats. Subsequently, there is a "proliferation" of macrophages in the basement membrane which continues as long the abnormal deposition of solutes continues. And, until vitamin C levels in the arteries normalize, abnormal deposits will continue to appear and macrophages will continue to proliferate and engulf the solutes, thereby continuing the relentless progression of atherosclerosis.

Section Two

Coronary Heart Disease Risk Factors and Vitamin C Deficiency

CHAPTER 3
High Blood Pressure and Vitamin C Deficiency

INADEQUATE VITAMIN C INITIATES HIGH BLOOD PRESSURE'S PLAQUE-BUILDING ACTIVITY

High blood pressure is a well-known risk factor for the development of atherosclerotic lesions in the arteries (Stamler et al., 1985; Hjerkinn et al., 2005; Kempler, 2005). What is not so well known is that high blood pressure does not act alone in contributing to arterial narrowings and blockages. Studies show that high blood pressure requires an accompanying lack of arterial vitamin C to initiate these damaging affects.

In order for an artery to maintain normal integrity over time in the presence of elevated (or even normal) blood pressure, the collagen content in all three layers of the blood vessel must be of optimal amount and quality. Sufficient vitamin C must be taken on a regular basis in order for this to take place (Blanck and Peterkofsky, 1975; Wendt et al., 1997; May and Qu, 2005).

As more fully discussed in Chapter 2, when vitamin C levels remain low long enough, the first change that begins to take place in the blood vessel is what is known as a "degenerative" change. Simply put, the microscopic picture of such tissue shows a lessening of structural organization, which includes a lessening in the quantity of collagen. Furthermore, the collagen that is still present can be expected to be mechanically inferior and not as strong as normal collagen. The degradation of collagen quality can occur even if the collagen was originally created in the presence of adequate vitamin C.

Lanman and Ingalls (1937) were able to show that the healed wounds in guinea pigs deprived of vitamin C had "greatly inferior tensile strength" compared to the healed wounds of animals given adequate vitamin C. Stolman et al. (1961) were able to show that normally formed collagen showed an early breakdown when vitamin C supplementation was withdrawn from guinea pigs.

Abt et al. (1959) were also able to show that vitamin C is essential not only for normal tissue healing, but also for the maintenance of previously formed scar tissue. Pirani and Levenson (1953) also found that scar tissue is more sensitive than normal connective tissue to the deficiency of vitamin C.

This finding directly implies that maintenance of the atherosclerotic, "scarred" blood vessel requires even more vitamin C to maintain its integrity, however impaired, than if it had developed normally in the presence of adequate amounts of vitamin C. The presence and quality of collagen is probably the most significant factor in determining how mechanically strong a healed wound, or a blood vessel, will be.

When there are abnormal amounts of mechanically inferior collagen in a given area of a blood vessel wall, some degree of break-

EXHIBIT 9

Plaque is a type of arterial scar tissue.

down and degeneration of the normal tissue structure can be expected to be one of the first detectable changes under the microscope.

Logically, if a normal vitamin C status could be regained at the point of early breakdown or degeneration of the collagen substructure of the blood vessel, a complete or near-complete healing of the blood vessel could be anticipated. However, when the levels of vitamin C remain low over a prolonged period of time, adequate amounts of quality collagen and other important proteins simply cannot be synthesized, and the body proceeds to compensate in the only way it can.

EXHIBIT 10

Even larger levels of vitamin C are essential for proper healing of damaged tissues and maintenance of scar tissue.

If no compensatory mechanism existed, the blood vessel would relentlessly continue its degeneration until it became so weak that it eventually failed, with progressive enlarging of the vessel's diameter (dilatation), leaking of blood, and/or frank rupture.

To prevent this ultimately lethal outcome, the body starts a compensatory mechanism known as a "proliferative" reaction. Simply put, without the normal amounts of quality collagen being present in the blood vessel wall the body has to find a way to strengthen the blood vessel wall. The body accomplishes this wall strengthening by stimulating intense cellular proliferation, typically with fibroblasts, in the intima and the immediately adjacent media.

As this cellular multiplication proceeds, the blood vessel wall physically thickens over areas that had been depleted of collagen, in the form of an evolving atherosclerotic plaque. This thickening is the body's way of focally fortifying the blood vessel wall in the absence of normal collagen formation, as the eventual consequence of vitamin C deficiency in that specific location.

Ironically, the mature fibrous plaque of atherosclerosis actually has a high concentration of collagen in it (Levene and Poole, 1962). As just discussed, in order to strengthen areas of collagen-deficient vessel walls, the body stimulates the mass production of fibroblasts.

Fibroblasts are the cells that produce collagen and these newly created cells start to cover areas of the internal surface of the arterial wall, putting them in direct contact with the blood flow. This proximity to the blood flow undoubtedly allows these newly created "collagen factories" to better grab circulating vitamin C than if they had to rely on the vitamin C penetrating the deeper reaches of the arterial wall. And, even while collagen production is increasing in the plaque itself, it still remains depleted in the arterial wall as long as overall vitamin C levels in the body remain depressed.

Crawford and Levene (1953) were able to demonstrate that the media of the arterial wall was physically thinned and decreased in mass, even when directly under an area of atherosclerotic thickening of the blood vessel wall. This supports the concept that deeper areas of the atherosclerotic blood vessel wall remain collagen-poor even when the compensatory fibrous thickenings atop such areas are collagen-rich.

Not surprisingly, the actual composition of the fibrous atherosclerotic thickening is variable, depending upon the variety of risk factors present. After the thickening is initiated by the cellular proliferation, more mature, obstructive blockages in the artery can then evolve in a number of different ways.

These advanced lesions are known as fibrous plaques, and they can subsequently become sites of hemorrhage, complete blood vessel blockage, and/or calcification. Furthermore, whenever there is the slightest degree of hemorrhage or even leakage of blood into an atherosclerotic plaque, further stimulation of fibroblastic growth can be anticipated, as the presence of hemoglobin is known to induce such growth (Baker, 1929). Certainly, it has been established that hemorrhage into a plaque (intraplaque) will lead to overall plaque progression and growth (Corti et al., 2004). This is likely one of the reasons why advanced atherosclerotic plaques are more difficult to completely reverse than early lesions.

Strongly supporting the concept that high blood pressure can initiate atherosclerosis and promote its continued development by overtaxing collagen-depleted blood vessels walls is the fact that advanced atherosclerosis does not typically develop in arteries within the heart (intramyocardial coronary arteries) (Cheng, 2000; Scher, 2000). An *intramyocardial coronary artery* is one that courses directly through the heart muscle itself.

The diseased coronary arteries that are the focus of a bypass surgery or a balloon angioplasty procedure are always "epicardial," meaning that they course over the exterior of the heart, with only their intramyocardial branches dipping into the heart muscle. This means that the epicardial coronary artery has only the resistance offered by the blood vessel wall itself to counter the ongoing burden/trauma of elevated blood pressure.

Consistent with this assertion is the fact that the distribution of atherosclerotic plaques in the epicardial coronary arteries is concentrated in the areas of highest physical stress, such as the points of bifurcation and branching (Thubrikar and Robicsek, 1995). The intramyocardial coronary artery, however, has the dense, strong heart muscle completely surrounding it. Even when such an artery is depleted of its normal content of collagen, the artery is not in danger of significant secondary dilatation, with subsequent weakening, leakage, and/or rupture. Because this danger does not exist, the body does not have the need to institute any compensatory measures to prevent it from happening,

EXHIBIT 11

High blood pressure can initiate and promote continued plaque build up by overtaxing collagen-depleted blood vessels.

and no significant cellular proliferative response sub-sequently develops, even though the intramyocardial coronary artery might be low on collagen as well. This is also supported by the fact that non-obstructive en-dothelial disease and early atherosclerosis can readily be found in intramyocardial arteries (Cooper and Hea-gerty, 1998; Cantin et al., 2002; Hu et al., 2005). How-ever, high-grade, fully evolved lesions do not typically develop in those vessels as they do in the epicardial coronary arteries. Therefore, it is reasonable to postu-late that high blood pressure is really only a significant risk factor for atherosclerosis when three conditions are met:

1) Vitamin C deficiency has been present for a long enough period of time,
2) The levels of collagen and other important structural proteins in the arterial walls are ad-equately depleted, and
3) No additional external support around the blood vessel wall is available, as with the epi-cardial coronary artery (Robicsek and Thubri-kar, 1994).

VITAMIN C DEFICIENCY SHOWN TO CAUSE AND SUSTAIN HIGH BLOOD PRESSURE

There is an additional reason high blood pres-sure needs a chronic vitamin C deficiency in order to express its full potential as a risk factor for atheroscle-rosis. Vitamin C deficiency has been shown to play an integral role in the actual causation and sustaining of high blood pressure (Bates et al., 1998; Fotherby et al.,

2000; May, 2000). Consistent with this, Galley et al. (1997) found that a combined antioxidant supplementation that included vitamin C was effective in reducing blood pressure. Furthermore, Duffy et al. (1999) demonstrated in a double-blind, placebo-controlled study that vitamin C was effective as a monotherapy in lowering the blood pressure of hypertensive patients. Studies have also shown that higher blood levels of vitamin C are clearly related to lower blood pressure in humans (Moran et al., 1993; Ness et al., 1996; Ness et al., 1997; Sakai et al., 1998).

EXHIBIT 12

High levels of vitamin C shown effective in lowering blood pressure in humans

By two seemingly independent mechanisms, then, vitamin C deficiency facilitates both the elevation of blood pressure itself as well as the susceptibility of the blood vessel wall to be damaged by that elevated pressure.

In addition, adequate vitamin C levels not only make the development of significantly high blood pressure unlikely, but normal levels of collagen in the blood vessel walls would probably render any blood pressure elevation of little or no consequence in the development of atherosclerosis. As a risk factor for atherosclerosis and coronary heart disease, then, high blood pressure appears to need a significant vitamin C deficiency for maximal effect.

CHAPTER 4

Inflammation and Vitamin C Deficiency

A PROBABLE MECHANISM FOR DELIVERING VITAMIN C TO DEFICIENT ARTERIES

Inflammation also appears to be a major player in the development, progression, and ultimate destabilization of atherosclerotic lesions, ultimately leading to the complete obstruction of an artery (Yu and Rifai, 2000; MacCallum, 2005; Boos and Lip, 2006).

Becker et al. (2001) and Corti et al. (2004) have noted that plaques prone to complications — such as sudden complete obstruction — contain large numbers of inflammatory cells, while stable plaques that have a lesser complication rate have less evidence of inflammation.

Inflammation is defined as a protective response to the injury or destruction of tissue, aiming to lessen the injuring agent and wall off (isolate) the affected area. In addition to causing other effects, inflammation also serves to attract white blood cells to the site of damage. While there are certainly multiple reasons why inflammation can be initiated, one possible reason that should be given consideration is that inflammation is also a mechanism that can assure a specific delivery of vitamin C to an injured site.

Evans et al. (1982) were able to demonstrate that different types of white blood cells can have anywhere

EXHIBIT 13

Cells associated with inflammation– white blood cells and macrophages– have up to 80 times more vitamin C than blood plasma.

from 25 to 80 times greater concentrations of vitamin C than that found in the blood plasma. Even in states of severe vitamin C deficiency, the white blood cells will still selectively concentrate what vitamin C is available. Also, macrophages are very common cells involved in inflammation, and the macrophages derive from white blood cells known as monocytes, which Evans et al. found to have the greatest vitamin C concentrations (80-fold concentration) of the blood cell components they tested.

Furthermore, Willis and Fishman (1955) have

EXHIBIT 14

Human arteries are commonly depleted of vitamin C, even in individuals who appear to be well-nourished.

documented that human arteries are commonly depleted of vitamin C, even in individuals who were "apparently well-nourished." They even found that localized depletions of vitamin C often existed in segments of arteries subjected to greater mechanical stress. Such

segments had already been identified as having been especially susceptible to the development of atherosclerosis in Chapter 3, which addresses hypertension as a risk factor.

Therefore, one explanation for the ongoing appearance of inflammation seen in atherosclerotic lesions is that the body is attempting to directly deliver vitamin C to the arterial areas most depleted of it via the white blood cells carrying the relatively greater amounts of vitamin C. Perhaps, at least for atherosclerosis, inflammation is only an attempt to keep local levels of vitamin C from getting even lower.

This concept of inflammation serving as a vitamin C delivery tool would also fit with the nature of the long-term inflammatory response seen in atherosclerosis, as inflammation does not typically appear for only a little while and then resolve in the absence of anti-inflammatory agents and measures.

The vitamin C deficiency persists in the atherosclerotic artery, and the inflammation may persist to some degree in an attempt to compensate for that deficiency. And, of course, the artery also suffers the long-term consequences of chronic inflammation from the body's attempts to deal with the shortage of vitamin C in the arterial tissue.

Even though such inflammation may be the body's way of getting more vitamin C to an atherosclerotic artery in the face of low body levels of vitamin C, it is also a factor that facilitates the further development of the arterial narrowing when it continues to persist unchecked.

Compensatory mechanisms that initially protect and facilitate healing will typically cause pathology when the compensatory process becomes chronic and unchecked (Licastro et al., 2005). Langlois et al. (2001) looked at patients with severe atherosclerosis in their legs, frequently finding the indicators of chronic inflammation and low vitamin C levels in the blood. They further suggested that the low vitamin C levels were probably directly related both to the presence of inflammation and the severity of the vascular disease.

Still further information supporting the notion that inflammation serves to draw vitamin C to the inflamed site comes from some research on the effects of insulin on inflammation. Dandona et al. (2001) were able to conclude from their research that insulin has a potent anti-inflammatory effect. Furthermore, they were able to demonstrate that insulin reduces

EXHIBIT 15

Insulin, a natural anti-inflammatory agent , transports vitamin C into inflamed cells which helps to neutralize the inflammation.

the cellular levels of some of the products of excess oxidation ("reactive oxygen species"), as well as the levels of several other substances known to promote inflammation. As insulin is now known to directly facilitate the transport of vitamin C into cells (Qutob et al., 1998; Rumsey et al., 2000), it may well be that this ability of insulin is the main reason for these observed lower levels of oxidation byproducts in these cells after insulin therapy.

In any event, it appears that the presence of more intracellular vitamin C helps to neutralize the products of inflammation inside those cells. This again implies that inflammation may well serve to attract vitamin C to inflamed tissues so that the inflammatory process, with its increased products of oxidation, will be ultimately "cooled off" and quenched by the increased cellular levels of vitamin C.

MANY IF NOT ALL CAUSES OF ARTERIAL INFLAMMATION DEPLETE VITAMIN C

Chronic inflammation in atherosclerosis, with an increased risk of heart attack from the total blockage of a heart artery, has also been related to the presence of chronic periodontal (gum and adjacent bone) disease (Beck et al., 1999; Muhlestein, 2000; Emingil et al., 2000). Similarly, periodontal disease has also been found to be associated with the development of carotid artery atherosclerosis (Soder et al., 2005).

EXHIBIT 16

Periodontal gum disease – a source of chronic arterial inflammation– linked to atherosclerosis

Such dental disease chronically releases bacteria and other infectious agents, as well as their associated toxins, from the mouth and gums into the blood. A similar effect will be consistently seen when any root canal-treated teeth are present (Meinig, 1996; Kulacz and Levy, 2002). When the dental disease goes unchecked or unaddressed, this seeding of microbes and toxins becomes chronic, and a popular target for these noxious agents is the readily accessible arterial wall. Once these agents

EXHIBIT 17

Dental disease and root canal-treated teeth release a continual flow of bacteria and toxins into the blood reach the arterial wall, vitamin C depletion can start or be further enhanced there.

Vitamin C is arguably the best and most versatile anti-microbial agent yet to be identified (Levy, 2002), and the lack of vitamin C in areas of developing atherosclerosis (Willis and Fishman, 1955) can significantly enhance the ability for microbes to continue to infect or colonize there.

EXHIBIT 18

A lack of the anti-microbial power of vitamin C enhances ability of microbes to infect and colonize arterial walls.

Even if the rest of the body is vitamin C-deficient and susceptible to infection as well, the blood vessels are the first tissues to deal with the microorganisms and toxins squeezed from infectious periodontal disease into the blood. Indeed, the DNA specific for multiple periodontal microbes/pathogens has been detected in atherosclerotic plaques (Hajishengallis et al., 2002). Such a microbe/toxin presence is yet another reason for the presence of chronic inflammation in arteries with developing atherosclerosis.

EXHIBIT 19

Microbial infection possibly a primary reason for chronic inflammation of the arterial wall.

Microbes from pockets of infection other than in the mouth can also chronically seed the blood vessel linings and promote chronic inflammation. Becker, et al (2001) also asserted the likelihood of infection being a primary reason for chronic inflammation of the arterial wall. Therefore, the lack of vitamin C can promote inflammation in the arteries both by allowing microbes to set up shop without too much of a fight, and by serving as an attraction to the inflammation process in order to have more vitamin C delivered to a depleted area when the body stores are low. Also, any microbe-associated toxins released into the blood from remote sites of infection will serve to accelerate the consumption of circulating vitamin C, keeping the levels of vitamin C in the arterial walls especially low, further facilitating the successful colonization of microbes there.

Infection, which will always have some component of associated inflammation, has long been observed to at least be associated with different forms of arterial disease. Klotz (1906 and 1906a) conducted experiments that indicated that some infections, including streptococcal ones, tended to stimulate cell proliferation in the intima and inner medial layers of the blood vessel, much like the "traditional" form of atherosclerosis.

EXHIBIT 20

Autopsies reveal certain microbial infections cause localized inflammation, swelling and death of arterial tissue.

In autopsy examinations, Weisel (1906 and 1906a) found that many other infections, such as diphtheria, scarlet fever, measles, chickenpox, pneumonia, influenza, and septicemia, induced almost purely a disease of the arterial media, with inflammation, swelling, and some death of arterial tissue. This is the same area of the blood vessel wall that Menten and King (1935) demonstrated to be affected most directly by diphtheria toxin.

It should also be noted that the rate of development of atherosclerosis in the face of infection can be very rapid. Willis (1953) noted infection in guinea pigs could produce identifiable atherosclerosis when they were fed a "full diet" and sick for only "a day or two." Willis (1957) also noted that the early lesions of atherosclerosis were completely reversible. He also showed that this reversibility could be achieved very quickly.

Until it becomes more chronic and entrenched, atherosclerosis appears to be a very dynamic process, and many people undoubtedly resolve a great number of minor or early atherosclerotic lesions before the lesions grow to a point that quick resolution is no longer feasible.

EXHIBIT 21

Some microbial infections can generate autoimmune reaction against components in arterial walls.

In addition to associated inflammation and infection-related toxins, infections can also contribute to the development of atherosclerosis by generating autoimmune reactions against components of the blood vessel wall (Kiechl et al., 2001; Leskov and Zatevakhim, 2005).

An autoimmune reaction occurs when the immune system directs itself against tissue sites that are altered by influences such as infections or toxins and no longer look "normal" to the immune system. Rather, the immune system looks at such altered tissue as "foreign," mobilizing antibodies and immune cells to attack this tissue as though it were an alien intruder. Such altered tissue sites capable of provoking an immune response have been demonstrated in atherosclerotic lesions by Wick et al. (1997).

Furthermore, autoimmune antibodies have been demonstrated to attack endothelial cells in culture (Mayr et al., 1999) and have been correlated with atherosclerotic disease in the carotid artery (Xu et al., 1999). Xu et al. (2000) have also demonstrated elevated levels of autoimmune antibodies in patients known to have atherosclerosis. Kleindienst et al. (1995) also outlined evidence that atherosclerosis commonly has an autoimmune component.

EXHIBIT 22

Individuals with autoimmune disease show increased prevalence of atherosclerosis.

It is now well-established that autoimmune disease is associated with an increased prevalence of atherosclerosis (de Leeuw et al., 2005; Doria et al., 2005; Frostegard, 2005). In addition to its many other functions and uses, vitamin C has also been shown to be effective in treating autoimmune disease (Kodama et al., 1994). It would seem, then, that the ability to lessen the intensity of an autoimmune reaction provoked by inflammation and/or infection is but one more reason why properly dosed vitamin C would be highly effective in the treatment of atherosclerosis.

Viral infections have also been specifically implicated in the development of atherosclerosis (Fabricant et al., 1978; Minick et al., 1979; Fabricant et al., 1983). A specific type of herpesvirus was inoculated into chickens that were fed either cholesterol-poor or cholesterol-rich diets. Two uninfected control groups were also followed. Atherosclerosis could not be induced in uninfected chickens, even when fed extra cholesterol.

On the other hand, infected chickens, whether with elevated or normal cholesterol levels, developed grossly visible lesions of atherosclerosis in the coronary arteries, the aorta, and the major branches off the aorta. Microscopically, the atherosclerotic lesions were found to closely resemble the lesions of chronic atherosclerosis in man. Blum et al. (2005) found that higher viral loads in patients infected with human immunodeficiency virus (HIV) were associated with poorer endothelial function, another condition felt to play an important role in the evolution of atherosclerosis.

It would seem prudent, then, to consider the possibility that many of the viral diseases faced by man must be considered as possible causes, aggravators and/or potentiators of the atherosclerotic process.

EXHIBIT 23

Vitamin C is the main effective defense against acute or chronic viral infections and the only definitive cure for many viral diseases

Other investigators have provided clear evidence of viruses promoting the development of atherosclerosis (Adam et al., 1987; Cunningham and Pasternak, 1988; Melnick et al., 1995; Eryol et al., 2005). Nicholson and Hajjar (1999) also offered evidence that herpes viruses may even serve as blood-clotting activators, perhaps playing a role in provoking the total arterial blockages often seen in the late stages of atherosclerosis. Furthermore, vitamin C has been proven to be the main effective defense against acute or chronic viral infections, and it remains the only therapy proven to definitively cure many viral diseases (Levy, 2002).

A state of vitamin C deficiency, then, can serve to both start and maintain the presence of atherosclerosis-inducing viruses in the body.

Even if inflammation is serving a role to attract more vitamin C to a depleted arterial wall, the inflammation itself, unless very acute and short-lived, is probably going to do more harm from its associated activities than good from any vitamin C delivered by the cells.

Becker et al. (2001) noted that the ongoing inflammatory process favors tissue degradation or breakdown. Even though acute inflammation is an essential part of normal healing, chronic inflammation more commonly works against definitive healing.

Some of the anti-cholesterol drugs known as statins are now being found to have anti-inflammatory activity and even antioxidant activity (Karatzis et al., 2005; Morita et al., 2005; Zieden and Olsson, 2005). These drugs appear to decrease the likelihood of cardiac death from atherosclerosis by more than just the mechanism of reducing elevated blood cholesterols.

EXHIBIT 24

High blood levels of C-reactive protein are associated with greater degrees of inflammation and greater risk of atherosclerosis

Ridker et al. (1999) demonstrated that the administration of one of the statin drugs, pravastatin, results in significantly lower levels of C-reactive protein. High blood levels of C-reactive protein are associated with greater degrees of inflammation and greater risk of atherosclerosis (Morrow and Ridker, 2000; Ilhan et al., 2005; Makita et al., 2005; Sun et al., 2005).

Also, C-reactive protein is frequently found to be deposited in atherosclerotic lesions (Sun et al., 2005). Ridker et al. (2001) later showed that another statin drug, cerivastatin, rapidly reduced C-reactive protein levels independent of its anti-cholesterol effects in 785 patients with elevated cholesterol levels. This lowering of C-reactive protein levels implies that cerivastatin also possesses significant anti-inflammatory properties.

Inflammation also appears to induce a significant portion of its harmful effects on blood vessels by inducing vasoconstriction, with the resulting narrowing of the caliber of the vessels. Furthermore, it has been shown that when this vasoconstriction was induced in healthy human volunteers, it could corrected by the administration of vitamin C intra-arterially (Pleiner et al., 2003).

Inflammation, by multiple mechanisms, appears to be a significant risk factor for atherosclerotic heart disease. Vitamin C deficiency appears to possibly help stimulate the inflammation process by the need to deliver more vitamin C to depleted areas. Also, vitamin C deficiency definitely helps other inducers of inflammation to take hold in the body, such as bacterial and viral infections, as well as the toxins and autoimmune reactions they often produce.

Finally, inflammation appears to induce a chronic vasoconstriction in arteries that can be prevented or reversed with adequate dosing of vitamin C. Inflammation in the blood vessel walls, then, appears to be another risk factor for atherosclerosis that is only of maximal significance in the face of a severe enough depletion of vitamin C in the body.

CHAPTER 5
Cholesterol and Vitamin C Deficiency

Abnormal levels and abnormal types of fats in the blood also play a role in the development of atherosclerosis. Also known as dyslipidemia, the most common type known to the public (and the doctors) is the elevation of blood cholesterol levels. High enough levels of cholesterol do result in the increased development of atherosclerosis, but such levels of cholesterol are not typically the initiators of the atherosclerotic process. Instead, cholesterol is just one of a number of substances that will readily deposit in an area of the artery where atherosclerosis has already begun. Other types of blood fat, such as triglycerides, chylomicrons, and some lipoproteins, can also promote atherosclerosis when they exist in high enough concentrations in the blood.

Multiple trials have demonstrated that lowering the cholesterol level through medical, dietary, or surgical means decreases the incidence of coronary heart disease and the chance of death (heart attack) from it (Leren, 1970; Coronary Drug Project Research Group, 1975; Carlson et al., 1977; Lipid Research Clinics Program, 1984; Frick et al., 1987; Dorr et al., 1978; Buchwald et al., 1990; Brophy et al., 2005).

Unfortunately, all of this research has caused both the medical professionals and the public to assign cholesterol elevation the role as a primary cause of heart disease. Cholesterol only adds to the development of atherosclerosis after the process has been initiated by degenerative arterial changes taking place because of vitamin C deficiency.

Simultaneously, as we shall see, the toxins left unneutralized by the vitamin C deficiency are also a primary reason why serum cholesterol levels are higher, with their greater likelihood of depositing in areas of developing atherosclerosis. Furthermore, the excess toxicity that is often associated with elevated cholesterol levels has its own direct and indirect effects in the causation of atherosclerosis.

EXHIBIT 25

Vitamin C deficiency can cause cholesterol accumulation in heart arteries even when cholesterol was not added to the diet.

Ginter (1978) found that vitamin C deficiency alone in the guinea pig would result in the development of atherosclerosis. Under conditions of vitamin C deficiency, he noted that cholesterol and triglycerides accumulated in the aorta, even without adding cholesterol to the diet. These changes were found to lead to a fairly classic picture of fully developed atherosclerosis. Willis (1953) had also documented that deficient dietary vitamin C could be the sole reason for the development of atherosclerosis in the guinea pig. Willis asserted that the atherosclerotic lesions in the guinea pig, simply deprived of sufficient vitamin C intake, appeared physically identical in form and structure to those lesions seen in human atherosclerosis. Willis also found that when the guinea pigs were fed increased amounts of cholesterol, injected vitamin C demonstrated a protective effect against the development of atherosclerosis.

EXHIBIT 26

Vitamin C deficiency identified as a sole cause of atherosclerosis in laboratory animals.

Similarly, Datey et al. (1968) found that vitamin C administration reduced the incidence and severity of atherosclerosis in rabbits fed a diet high in cholesterol and hydrogenated fat. Ginter further noted that the simultaneous intake of additional cholesterol by the vitamin C-deprived guinea pigs did accelerate the development of atherosclerosis. It would appear from this evidence that the arterial changes that result from vitamin C deficiency make it easier for cholesterol and fats, whether elevated in the blood or not, to deposit in the blood vessel walls.

EXHIBIT 27

Administration of vitamin C reduces incidence and severity of atherosclerosis in cholesterol-fed animals.

Duff (1935) noted that elevated cholesterol levels alone were unlikely to result in atherosclerosis. Rather, he proposed that "local alterations" in the blood vessel walls were necessary to allow the deposition of cholesterol there.

This predisposition for cholesterol deposition was noted in Chapter 2 and involves the chemistry of the basement membrane in which the endothelial cells of the artery are embedded. When enough vitamin C is present, the basement membrane is well polymerized and gel-like, and when a significant vitamin C deficiency is present, the basement is poorly polymerized and watery. A watery basement membrane, secondary to vitamin C deficiency, appears necessary for any cholesterol or fat deposition to take place in this area of the blood vessel wall.

EXHIBIT 28

Cholesterol deposition in the arteries does not begin unless there is a prior injury to the blood vessel.

Duff also noted that some form of injury to the blood vessel was needed to initiate cholesterol deposition. Whenever an area of the blood vessel is injured to any degree, this is usually accompanied by at least a localized deficiency of vitamin C.

Willis and Fishman (1955) found that localized depletions of vitamin C were typically found in segments of arteries subjected to increased mechanical stress, which is a form of injury. This localized vitamin C deficiency can then allow the early cholesterol deposition in atherosclerosis to proceed in a very localized, focal manner in the affected basement membrane areas of the blood vessel wall.

Taylor et al. (1957) showed that a deliberate freezing injury to the artery in monkeys with high cholesterol levels appeared to "telescope into a few weeks" the development of atherosclerotic lesions that took several years to develop in humans. Although it was not measured, it would be reasonable to assume that the injured artery quickly became depleted of vitamin C as well.

Even today many clinicians and researchers consider atherosclerosis to be a "one-way" or irreversible process. Multiple researchers have demonstrated otherwise. Without addressing the vitamin C status, Taylor et al. (1961) found that cholesterol and fats are taken up by the blood vessel walls when serum cholesterol levels exceed 250 mg% (milligrams per 100 milliliters), and that they are "apparently resorbed" back from the blood vessel walls when serum cholesterol levels are below 200 mg%.

EXHIBIT 29

Cholesterol deposits in blood vessels shown to be reabsorbed by blood when blood level of cholesterol is below 200.

Horlick and Katz (1949) were able to show that atherosclerotic lesions induced in chicks by excessive cholesterol feeding were noted to clearly regress when the cholesterol feeding was discontinued. Since the chick is one of the great majority of animals that synthesizes its own vitamin C, internal vitamin C production may well be accelerating the resolution of the arterial lesions. Horlick and Katz noted a range of responses, with some lesions showing less stainable fat but more fibrosis when cholesterol feeding was discontinued, indicating advanced atherosclerotic lesions would not completely resolve under such circumstances. However, they also noted some animals that demonstrated virtually a "complete remission" of the atherosclerotic changes, whether viewed grossly or microscopically.

Anitschkow (1928 and 1933), one of the first investigators to look at the response of arterial lesions to the cessation of cholesterol feeding (in rabbits), described a gradual loss of lipids (fats) from atherosclerotic plaques. He also emphasized that the process was slow, noting that the evolution of a lipid-rich plaque into a plaque composed primarily of fibrous tissue took two to three years.

Interestingly, however, Horwitz and Katz noted that the rate of regression of lesions in the chicken was much greater than in the rabbit. This observation could possibly relate to the amounts of vitamin C available during the healing period, as all animals that can make their own vitamin C do not do so with equal efficiency. Undoubtedly, the amount of vitamin C available to the blood vessel wall, how far advanced the atherosclerotic lesion is and how much circulating cholesterol and fats are present in the blood are all significant determinants as to both the reversibility of the lesion and the length of time needed to achieve that reversibility.

Wilens (1947) was also able to indirectly help to demonstrate the importance of lipid and cholesterol levels in the maintenance of atherosclerotic disease of the blood vessels. In autopsy examinations, he was able to demonstrate that there was a "high incidence of severe atherosclerosis" in obese individuals, who often have higher lipid and cholesterol levels. Conversely, with individuals who had been subjected to "protracted undernutrition" even moderate changes of atherosclerosis were "seldom observed." Lipid and cholesterol levels will typically drop in such individuals.

While such a study does not address the role of vitamin C in such undernourished individuals, it does indicate that starvation will tend to pull cholesterol and lipids back out of atherosclerotic plaques. This finding alone clearly demonstrates that atherosclerosis is not irreversible.

Indeed, in radioactive isotope research on the atherosclerotic lesions of rabbits, cholesterol already present in the lesions has been demonstrated to be subject to continuous turnover, far from a simple static, cumulative process (Newman and Zilversmit, 1962).

EXHIBIT 30

Vitamin C retards penetration of cholesterol into blood vessels and increases release of cholesterol already present in those vessels.

Zaitsev et al. (1964) also looked at the movement of radioactively-tagged cholesterol in rabbits. They found that the effects of vitamin C on atherosclerosis resulted in less cholesterol penetration into the blood vessel along with increased release of cholesterol already in the blood vessel.

In order to fully appreciate much of the animal research on atherosclerosis, it is also critical to realize that animals can be induced to develop atherosclerosis by a mechanism and sequence not usually seen in humans. Lindsay and Chaikoff (1966) noted that atherosclerosis experimentally induced in animals without the assistance of a vitamin C deficiency evolved quite differently from human atherosclerosis.

However, they also noted that the atherosclerotic changes in the blood vessels of certain primates having the disease naturally were "similar, if not identical" to those changes seen in man. Lindsay and Chaikoff also noted that the degree of cholesterol infiltration in the blood vessels of primates is generally less than that seen in man. These differences can be readily explained by the greater toxin loads generally faced by man, such as from dental sources (Huggins and Levy, 1999), with corresponding higher chronically circulating cholesterol levels.

This correlation between toxins and elevated cholesterol levels will be discussed later in this chapter. Also, the primates as a group ingest much more vitamin C in their diets than humans as a group. Furthermore, Lindsay and Chaikoff noted that the naturally occurring form of atherosclerosis in animals had substantial microscopic differences compared to the artificially induced forms of atherosclerosis provoked by various efforts to increase blood cholesterol and other blood fats.

Lindsay and Chaikoff also noted that the natural form of atherosclerosis was initiated by a degenerative change in the intima of the blood vessel wall, followed secondarily by a proliferative fibrotic reaction. In other words, the initial change, degeneration, is itself an arterial stress that results in the compensatory response of cellular proliferation and fibrosis. This is the same sequence of events seen with the chronic depletion of vitamin C.

However, in the cholesterol-feeding forms of induced atherosclerosis, the "overdose" of cholesterol results in immune cells (macrophages) in the blood vessel walls taking up the excess cholesterol. Since a high enough level of cholesterol seems to have its own toxicity (Ginter, 1975), this macrophage response is very possibly a compensatory immune-mediated response to lessen the acute toxicity of the excess cholesterol. After enough of these macrophages have taken up enough cholesterol, this excessive presence of stuffed macrophages is also interpreted by the body as another arterial stress, and a proliferation of cells with secondary fibrosis can then result.

Mann et al. (1953) induced such lesions in cholesterol-fed monkeys. Basically, the abnormal amounts of cholesterol have to go somewhere, and the endothelial surfaces of the arterial walls are the first areas contacted. In fact, Shaffer (1970) noted that such cholesterol feeding to experimental animals is accompanied by "extreme" depositing of cholesterol and lipids throughout the body, not just in the blood vessels. And in vitamin C-supplemented rabbits, Beetens et al., (1984) were able to demonstrate, after only a few weeks of a cholesterol-rich diet, a clearly lessened degree of intimal thickening and lipid infiltration.

EXHIBIT 31

Animals fed high doses of cholesterol show rapid reductions of vitamin C in plasma and cells.

High doses of cholesterol, in exerting the toxic effects described by Ginter (1975), appear to rapidly metabolize vitamin C just like any other toxin or toxic effect. Dent et al. (1951) were able to demonstrate that feeding cholesterol to rabbits and other animals results in a drop in the vitamin C levels in both plasma and cells. Booker et al. (1957) achieved a similar depression of the vitamin C levels in rabbits and guinea pigs given a continual administration of cholesterol.

These findings seem to indicate that the technique of overfeeding cholesterol to laboratory animals also serves to promptly induce a vitamin C deficiency as well. This rapidly induced vitamin C deficiency allows the basement membrane behind the endothelial cells to allow or facilitate the deposition of the cholesterol and blood fat as the glycoproteins degenerate and the consistency becomes watery. In any event, the atherosclerosis that is eventually developed through either "natural" or artificial mechanisms is comparable enough that the results of animal atherosclerosis experimentation can generally be used to help understand human atherosclerosis.

Vitamin C interacts with and affects cholesterol metabolism in a number of ways. Turley et al. (1976) reviewed the literature and concluded that chronic but latent vitamin C deficiency leads to increased blood levels of cholesterol. Ginter (1973) found that high levels of vitamin C lower the cholesterol concentration in both the serum and the liver in guinea pigs. Sitaramayya and Ali (1962) also found that in both rats and guinea pigs the administration of vitamin C prevented the cholesterol level in the blood from increasing after cholesterol feeding.

Ginter (1975a) and Ginter et al. (1971) also found in guinea pigs that low levels of vitamin C reduce the rate of metabolic transformation of cholesterol into bile acids, its principal breakdown product, leading to increased levels of cholesterol.

In rabbits, Sadava et al. (1982) were able to show that supplemental vitamin C can protect against elevated blood cholesterol even when cholesterol is administered by injection to rabbits.

Banerjee and Singh (1958) found that scurvy-stricken guinea pigs had a significant increase in total body cholesterol levels, again reflecting the pivotal role of vitamin C in maintaining normal cholesterol metabolism. Maeda et al. (2000) similarly found that mice rendered unable to synthesize vitamin C, effectively a "guinea pig equivalent," demonstrated higher total cholesterol levels and lower HDL-cholesterol levels with lower plasma vitamin C levels.

EXHIBIT 32

Relatively low daily doses of vitamin C for 47 days significantly reduced cholesterol levels in humans tested.

Cholesterol levels and vitamin C levels appear similarly related in man. Ginter et al. (1970) gave only 300 mg of vitamin C daily for 47 days to a group of individuals over 40 years of age. A significant decrease in cholesterol levels was seen, and the effect was especially pronounced in individuals with cholesterol levels above 240 mg%. These individuals had an average drop of 34 mg% in their levels.

Ginter et al. (1977) later showed that 1,000 mg of vitamin C daily for a full year had a comparable effect on cholesterol levels. Ginter et al. (1978) also looked at diabetic patients and found that 500 mg of vitamin C daily over the course of a year resulted in striking cholesterol drops, ranging from 40 mg% to 100 mg% in a majority of the patients.

Another dietary fat, triglycerides, also showed a moderate decline with the vitamin C administration given to Ginter's patients just noted above. The metabolism of triglycerides is also subject to some regulation by vitamin C.

Immediately after eating, the plasma will often be clouded by an increased content of triglycerides. Lipoprotein lipase (LPL), an enzyme also known as the clearing factor, serves to promptly metabolize these triglycerides and clear the clouded plasma.

Sokoloff et al. (1966) found that vitamin C not only lowered the levels of cholesterol and triglycerides in rabbits and rats with high cholesterol levels, it also enhanced the activity of LPL (the clearing factor) while minimizing the development of atherosclerotic lesions. They also demonstrated that in 50 of 60 patients with increased cholesterol levels and/or heart disease 2,000 to 3,000 mg of vitamin C daily increased the average LPL activity by 100% and decreased the average triglyceride level by 50% to 70%. As Weinhouse and Hirsch (1940) demonstrated that cholesterol is not the only fatty substance that accumulates in atherosclerotic plaques, it would seem that the favorable effects that

EXHIBIT 33

Most patients taking 3,000 mg of vitamin C/day increased LPL levels by 100% and decreased triglyceride levels by 50% to 70%.

vitamin C has on the activity level of LPL also plays an integral role in minimizing or reversing the development of atherosclerotic lesions.

THE IMPORTANT TOXIN-FIGHTING ABILITIES OF CHOLESTEROL

Vitamin C also relates to cholesterol levels in the body in another extremely important, although indirect fashion. The scientific literature reveals an abundance of evidence indicating that cholesterol serves as a primary neutralizer or inactivator of a wide array of toxic substances in both animal and human studies (Figueiredo et al., 2003; Park et al., 2005).

Alouf (1981 and 2000) reported the ability of cholesterol to neutralize a large number of different bacterial toxins capable of causing direct cellular damage. Chi et al. (1981) published data that indicated elevated serum cholesterols seemed to be a marker of, if not a direct response to, a variety of toxic exposures.

EXHIBIT 34

Cholesterol neutralizes a large number of bacterial toxins capable of causing direct cellular damage.

Watson and Kerr (1975) noted that the cell membrane-bound cholesterol in the arterial walls could not only bind bacterial toxins, it could also end up being a focus of reactive immune activity and act as one more agent promoting atherosclerotic damage.

Increased toxic pesticide exposures have been noted to correlate with increased cholesterol levels in the population of people exposed (Bloomer et al.,

1977). Similarly, in rabbits exposed to lead, Tarugi et al. (1982) found a "striking elevation" of cholesterol to result. Yousef et al., (2003) showed that aflatoxin exposure increased cholesterol levels in rabbits, and that vitamin C administration significantly lowered those cholesterol levels and clinically alleviated the harmful effects of the exposure.

EXHIBIT 35

Exposure to toxins and pesticides increases cholesterol levels.

Finally, Huggins and Levy (1999) have repeatedly observed significant drops in serum cholesterol levels in patients who have had mercury amalgams, root canals, and other sources of heavy metal and infective toxicity removed from their mouths.

EXHIBIT 36

Patients show significant serum cholesterol reductions after removal of dental toxicity.

Overall, then, it appears that one of cholesterol's many functions in the body is that of a relatively nonspecific toxin neutralizer and/or inactivator. Because of this role, cholesterol levels appear to be routinely elevated in conditions of increased toxin exposure, representing another of the body's compensatory mechanisms that, left unchecked, can cause its own significant harm by accelerating atherosclerosis.

The toxin-inactivating effects of cholesterol notwithstanding, vitamin C still appears to be the ultimate toxin neutralizer and inactivator. When higher levels of vitamin C are present to neutralize whatever toxins are present, cholesterol levels will not have to rise (and do not rise) in order to protect against those toxins. The cholesterol levels will end up remaining in the normal range. However, chronically low cholesterol levels generally leave much toxicity unneutralized even when vitamin C intake would otherwise be adequate. In these cases, any compensatory increase in cholesterol will then be one of the body's remaining best defense mechanisms against that toxicity, in the absence of more vigorously supplemented vitamin C.

Therefore, in addition to high cholesterol levels promoting atherosclerosis by being available for direct deposition into the developing lesions, high cholesterols are also directly indicative that there are abnormally high levels of chronic toxin exposure. Such toxins will have their own direct effects on promoting atherosclerosis, as well as their indirect effects by serving to much more rapidly metabolize whatever vitamin C is present in the body. This increased metabolism of vitamin C can both maintain and worsen the vitamin C deficiency that first initiated the atherosclerotic process.

Further evidence that cholesterol exerts this very important protective role against toxicity comes from studies that demonstrate an increased incidence of cancer or death from cancer in individuals with abnormally low cholesterol levels (Kark et al., 1980;

EXHIBIT 37

Patients with abnormally low cholesterol levels have increased incidence of cancer and death from cancer.

Williams et al., 1981; Kagan et al., 1981; Stemmermann et al., 1981; Keys et al., 1985; Gerhardsson et al., 1986; Schatzkin et al., 1987; Knekt et al., 1988; Isles et al., 1989; Cowan et al., 1990).

More recently, it was demonstrated specifically that low levels of high density lipoprotein cholesterol (the "good" cholesterol) was significantly related to an increased risk of cancer (Mainous et al., 2005). One straightforward explanation for this correlation is that chronically low cholesterol levels leave significant chronic toxin exposures unneutralized, and cancer is but one of the consequences one would expect from such persistent toxicity. Furthermore, a number of the cholesterol-lowering trials that have demonstrated less heart deaths with lower cholesterol levels have shown almost equally significant increases in deaths from a number of other causes, including suicide, accidents, and violence (Golomb, 1998; Golomb et al., 2000).

Supporting this concept, Marcinko et al. (2005) showed that psychiatric patients with violent suicidal attempts had significantly lower cholesterol levels than patients with non-violent suicide attempts and the control subjects.

EXHIBIT 38

Psychiatric patients with violent suicidal attempts had significantly lower cholesterol levels.

Unneutralized chronic toxicity, such as from a heavy metal like mercury, commonly produces such clinical symptoms as depression, impaired nervous and muscular function, irritability, and emotional instability. Depression from unneutralized toxicity can eventually result in suicide if the toxicity remains unaddressed, and the toxic effect continues to escalate.

Greater degrees of unneutralized toxicity will reliably lead to greater unchecked irritability and emotional instability, a condition that would facilitate a greater chance of violent suicide or death from violence. Similarly, progressive loss of muscle function and coordination can eventually result in fatal accidents, particularly in cars.

Cholesterol-lowering agents certainly appear to help stabilize the progression of or even help reverse atherosclerosis (Brown et al., 1990; Brown et al., 1993; Brown et al., 1993a; Brown et al., 1993b). However, they also leave the body with less protection from a continuous assault of environmental toxins, and susceptible individuals can end up dying from what might initially seem to be completely unrelated circumstances that do not "require" a logical explanation.

Interestingly, a similar clinical profile to that of mercury toxicity can result from almost any chronic, low-grade toxin exposure, although some toxins might have one or more other relatively unique clinical characteristics.

Virtually all toxins rapidly and significantly consume vitamin C, and the resulting vitamin C deficiency can make the effects of any toxins remaining in the body more significant, helping to give the common clinical picture of many different chronic toxin exposures, which is very similar to that described above for mercury toxicity.

In other words, all toxins can have direct toxic effects on target tissues, and they can indirectly result in many other nonspecific symptoms by virtue of the rapid consumption of the body's vitamin C stores. Furthermore, the rapid destruction of vitamin C by toxins will make the subsequent exposure to new toxins of much greater clinical consequence.

Ginter (1975) points out another interesting relationship between vitamin C and cholesterol. In rabbits and rats, which can synthesize vitamin C (unlike the guinea pig), a forced high cholesterol diet results in the accumulation of vitamin C in the liver and kidneys, with a dramatic increase in vitamin C excreted in the urine. This forced ingestion of large amounts of cholesterol seems to indicate that the animals respond to this cholesterol dosing by making more vitamin C.

Ginter (1975) suggests that this response to exceptionally high dietary cholesterol is like the response of any vitamin C-synthesizing animal to a toxin. Ginter also points out that excessive cholesterol has toxic effects on the rodent liver. This observation helps to explain why increased dietary cholesterol reduces tissue levels of vitamin C in guinea pigs (Ginter, 1970).

By whatever mechanism, high enough cholesterol doses are perceived by the organism as toxic, and vitamin C stores are promptly depleted. High cholesterol levels apparently increase demands for vitamin C because of the direct toxic effect of the high levels, as well as by the presence of the toxin(s) that the excess cholesterol is attempting to neutralize.

It would appear that elevated cholesterol levels can often routinely be normalized with the administration of vitamin C, unless the amounts of toxicity are so overwhelming that ordinary doses of vitamin C will not suffice and significant toxicity remains for the cholesterol to neutralize. Such extraordinary toxin exposures will be seen where there is a very large amount of industrial environmental toxin exposure, as from living downwind from a chemical factory.

Much more commonly, however, the toxic by-products of anaerobic bacterial metabolism generated in root canal-treated teeth are overwhelming to the body and virtually impossible to completely neutralize on a regular basis around-the-clock. The degree of toxicity found with such anaerobic bacterial metabolism is akin to and on the same magnitude as that of botulism.

Botulism toxin is currently regarded as one of the most potent toxins ever discovered. Root canal-treated teeth will routinely produce toxicity in a manner very similar to that seen when the botulism bacteria are unwittingly admitted into an oxygen-deprived environment, as is seen when they are accidentally trapped in a vacuum-packed can of food. The subsequent loss of oxygen in the can makes otherwise harmless bacteria highly toxic. In the root canal-treated tooth, bacteria from the mouth also become highly toxic when they settle in the oxygen-deprived environment of this pulpless tooth, which happens routinely.

The consistent toxicity of root canals is very well-documented, although not widely recognized or accepted (Meinig, 1996; Huggins and Levy, 1999; Kulacz and Levy, 2002). It is also a fact that is emotionally, although not

EXHIBIT 39

The consistent toxicity of root canals is well documented although not widely recognized or accepted.

scientifically, contested by the many dentists who routinely apply root canal treatments to their patients.

Willis et al. (1954) demonstrated that a majority of patients given only 500 mg of vitamin C orally three times a day had objective evidence of regression of atherosclerotic narrowings on follow-up angiography (X-rays of dye injected into the blood vessels). This regression was seen after a vitamin C administration period ranging from two to six months. A few patients showed no changes on follow-up, and a few patients showed detectable worsening of their arterial narrowings.

It is also very significant to note that any given patient showed the same changes in all lesions, i.e., improvement, worsening, or no change. No patient showed one lesion improving while another was narrowing further. These findings not only support the concept that vitamin C alone can reverse atherosclerosis, they also indicate the need for an adequate dosage of vitamin C to consistently achieve positive effects.

It is highly likely that the few patients who showed continued progression of their atherosclerotic lesions had ongoing toxin levels that 1,500 mg of vitamin C daily was simply incapable of significantly neutralizing. Those who showed no progression would appear to have been taking just enough vitamin C to neutralize daily toxicity without enough remaining to initiate significant vessel wall healing.

Any patient with a root canal-treated tooth, dead or infected tooth, or enough gum infection (periodontal disease) can be expected to have a daily toxin exposure

that would be little affected or insignificantly neutralized by a dose of only 1,500 mg vitamin C daily. Any
disease secondary to that toxicity would be expected to
proceed with little or no significant hindrance, just as
witnessed by Willis in the few patients whose atherosclerosis continued to progress even with the supplemented vitamin C.

Spittle (1971), after observing no recurrent heart
attacks or strokes in 60 patients given from 1 to 3 grams
of vitamin C daily over a 30-month period, asserted
that atherosclerosis is likely "a long-term deficiency
(or negative balance) of vitamin C, which permits cholesterol levels to build up in the arterial system, and
results in changes in other fractions of the fats."

Repeating the studies of Willis and Spittle with
a much higher oral dose of vitamin C (say, 6,000 to
12,000 mg daily), along with periodic intravenous
vitamin C administrations and the proper removal of
all root canal-treated teeth and other sources of dental
toxicity would likely show even more dramatic clinical
responses and lesion reversals in even a larger majority
of the patients treated.

As noted earlier, more cancer
is seen with lower cholesterol levels, which are indicative of higher
unneutralized toxin levels. Issels
(1999) specialized in the treatment
of cancer, finding that 98% of his
adult cancer patients had between

> **EXHIBIT 40**
>
> **Cancer doctor
> finds that 98% of
> his patients had
> between two and
> ten "dead teeth,"
> most of which were
> root canal-treated
> teeth.**

two and ten "dead teeth." Commonly, these were root
canal-treated teeth, which Issels also considered to be

dead and highly toxic. Such a high correlation between cancer and infective dental toxicity as typified by root canal-treated teeth is but one indication of how toxic such teeth can be, and of how difficult it is to maintain good health of any kind, cardiovascular or otherwise, as long as such teeth remain in the mouth.

Proper extraction of root canals and other infected teeth (with appropriate cleaning of the socket) is currently the only way to eliminate this very large source of chronic toxicity (Meinig, 1996; Levy and Huggins, 1996).

Two other substances that help to reverse and/or prevent atherosclerosis by their interactions with cholesterol metabolism deserve some elaboration here as well. The administration of chondroitin sulfates and of polyunsaturated lecithins has been shown to help stabilize atherosclerosis and sometimes reverse it. Both of these substances have biochemical interactions with vitamin C that play significant roles in allowing these substances to have their positive effects in the reversal or prevention of the development of atherosclerosis.

CHONDROITIN SULFATE, ATHEROSCLEROSIS, CHOLESTEROL, AND VITAMIN C

Chondroitin sulfate (CS) is a general term referring to a group of substances that have a large number of different biological effects, many of which either directly or indirectly reduce an individual's likelihood of developing atherosclerosis. CS is referred to in a number of different ways in the medical textbooks and the medical literature, which can be a bit confusing when trying to figure out what different groups of researchers are trying to say. Also referred to as acid mucopolysaccharides or glycosaminoglycans, CS is an important constituent of the ground substance of connective tissues. The importance of an intact ground substance (or basement membrane) in preventing the earliest manifestations of atherosclerosis in the artery wall was discussed in Chapter 2. While the relationship of CS and vitamin C is not clear-cut, it does appear that optimal quality of CS in the body for its optimal function does require the presence of optimal amounts of vitamin C.

Boumans and Mier (1970) found that guinea pigs with scurvy had a lower CS content in the connective tissue. It would appear that this decreased CS synthesis in scurvy is due to multiple factors, however, as vitamin C alone does not strongly stimulate CS synthesis (Kofoed and Robertson, 1966).

However, Edward and Oliver (1983), examining the degree of sulfur content of CS in human cells in culture, found that vitamin C appeared to increase the degree of sulfation in the CS, even though the net synthesis of CS was not increased.

It will be shown later in this chapter that the more CS is sulfated, the more positive are its overall biological effects. In other words, from a therapeutic point of view, vitamin C may not increase the overall quantity of CS in cells, but it does increase the quality (sulfate content) of the CS in exerting its beneficial effects on this substance. In support of these findings of

Edward and Oliver, Hatanaka and Egami (1976) earlier found that vitamin C bound to sulfate may very well be a critical substance in the incorporation of sulfate into chondroitin sulfate. Just as vitamin C can readily donate electrons in its pivotal role as an antioxidant, it also appears capable of binding sulfate groups and transferring (or donating) them to suitable acceptor molecules. Recently, Boskey et al. (2001) found that the vitamin C-sulfate complex causes an increased incorporation of sulfate into cartilage, further supporting the thesis that vitamin C may be very important in sulfate metabolism.

The vitamin C-sulfate complex has been shown to have another positive property. Verlangieri and Mumma (1973) were able to demonstrate that the sulfated form of vitamin C was able to increase the fecal excretion of cholesterol sulfate in rats by approximately 50-fold. Non-sulfated vitamin C only increased the excretion of cholesterol sulfate two-fold. This increased excretion would likely be a positive factor in the reduction of atherosclerosis. Their data also served to show that cholesterol, like chondroitin sulfate noted above, was another substance to which the sulfate in the vitamin C-sulfate complex could be transferred.

Clearly, the vitamin C-sulfate complex appears to have certain effects on cholesterol metabolism that are more pronounced than vitamin C alone. Several investigators have demonstrated that vitamin C and a vitamin C-sulfate complex have roughly comparable effects on lipid metabolism and atherosclerosis in guinea pigs, rabbits, rats, and mice (Finamore et al., 1976; Hayashi et al., 1976; Hayashi et al., 1978).

In the guinea pigs the sulfated vitamin C was also seen to help restore depleted levels of vitamin C. Overall, much less research on vitamin C bound to other substances has been done relative to the research done on vitamin C alone. However, such research could prove to be very helpful in maximizing the understanding of how vitamin C works, as well as understanding how its supplemental and medicinal actions might be optimized.

Murata (1962) reported that the anti-atherosclerotic properties of CS were more pronounced when the CS had a higher sulphur (or sulfate) content. Also, CS with a high sulphur content has been shown to inhibit several enzymes that can break down collagen and proteoglycans (Burkhardt and Ghosh, 1987).

Recall that proteoglycans are important in maintaining a healthy ground substance, the breakdown of which probably represents the beginning step of atherosclerosis. Any substance that can inhibit the breakdown of these vital proteoglycans would seem to be a positive nutrient.

Nakazawa et al. (1969) worked with two types of CS, chondroitin sulfate A (CSA) and chondroitin sulfate C (CSC). Their assays showed that their CSC had a higher sulfur content than their CSA. A similar difference in the sulfur contents of CSA and CSC was found by Izuka et al. (1968).

Furthermore, Nakazawa et al. (1969) demonstrated that their CSC also showed more striking positive effects than CSA on the atherosclerotic patients given these agents. Improvements in the electrocardiograms and prolongations of the times taken for the blood to clot were both more striking when the treating agent was CSC rather CSA.

Keeping the above comments in mind, it also appears that the amount of sulfate contained in CS appears to directly relate to its ability to inhibit the uptake of low density lipoproteins (LDL) in the arterial wall (Day et al., 1975). They found that CSC was significantly more effective than CSA in the inhibition of LDL uptake by the arterial wall, even though the CSA was still clearly of benefit in achieving this effect.

Recall that high density lipoprotein (HDL) is associated with the transport of cholesterol out of the arterial wall, while LDL is associated with the transport of cholesterol into the arterial wall. Therefore, inhibiting the uptake of LDL into the arterial wall also inhibits the uptake of cholesterol into the arterial wall. And although CS is not absolutely dependent upon vitamin C for its synthesis and function, it appears that optimal amounts of vitamin C assure that the CS is of optimal quality (highest sulfate content) for the optimal exertion of its anti-atherosclerotic properties. Vitamin C appears to support the formation of the vital components of the ground substance (noted earlier), while helping to increase the sulfate content of another substance (CS).

In addition to other improved benefits, this CS with a higher sulfate content helps prevent those essential elements of the ground substance from being broken down. Increased formation of the essential components of the ground substance along with a lessened breakdown of those substances together translates to a healthier ground substance, which is critical in blocking the first step of atherosclerosis.

One type of CS, chondroitin sulfate A (CSA), has been reported by Morrison (1971) to have the following significant biological properties:

- The ability to positively affect the metabolism of lipids (Morrison et al., 1963) and to more generally stimulate cellular metabolism (Morrison et al., 1965) in human tissue cultures,
- The ability to increase the rate of turnover of fatty acids at the cellular level,
- Anti-inflammatory effects in connective tissue,
- Anticoagulant (lessened blood clotting) effects in human studies (Izuka et al., 1968; Nakazawa et al., 1969),
- The ability to increase the development of new blood vessels (collateral circulation) in the hearts of rats with coronary artery atherosclerosis,
- Increased healing and repair activity after the complete blockage of heart arteries in rats, and
- Directly observed anti-atherosclerosis effects in monkeys with naturally occurring atherosclerosis (Morrison et al., 1966).

Note that even though Morrison described the above properties as belonging to CSA, CSC, with its higher sulfur content than CSA, should be expected to manifest all of these properties at least as well as CSA, if not better.

The interaction of the above properties of CSA can certainly help to explain its anti-atherosclerotic effects. In rats, Morrison et al. (1972) were able to demonstrate a significant ability of CSA to prevent atherosclerotic lesions from developing in rats fed a high-cholesterol diet, even though plasma cholesterol levels were not reduced by the therapy. Similarly, Matsushima et al. (1987) were able to show that CSC could suppress the development of atherosclerosis in rabbits fed a high-cholesterol diet, although the CSC administrations did lower plasma cholesterol levels.

This variable effect that CS has on cholesterol levels while consistently having an anti-atherosclerotic effect strongly implies that the primary effect of CS on cholesterol metabolism relates to its deposition and turnover of cholesterol in the arterial wall, not what maintains cholesterol levels in the blood.

In humans, Nakazawa and Murata (1975) reported on the effects of oral administration of CS on atherosclerotic subjects and on control subjects over a four-year period. Over twice as many deaths occurred in the control group, even though the average age of the heart patients in the treated group was higher than the average age of the subjects in the control group.

Morrison (1971) also found that CSA was a very effective agent in reducing the complications of heart disease. He found that chronic heart patients who were not given CSA had six-fold more clinical episodes related to narrowing or blockage of heart arteries than the group of chronic heart patients who were given CSA over a four-year study period.

Earlier, Morrison (1968) not only found that CSA had positive effects on the heart patients he treated, he also found that doses of CSA ranging from 1,500 mg to 10,000 mg daily over a period ranging from one to two years were well tolerated, without any toxic effects being noted.

Morrison (1968), in addition to demonstrating the positive effects of CSA on patients with atherosclerotic heart disease, noted that both the aging process and the presence of atherosclerosis are associated with decreased levels of CSA and CSC in the arterial wall, while other acid mucopolysaccharides, namely chondroitin sulfate B (CSB), heparitin sulfate, and dermatan sulfate, tend to increase in concentration in the arterial wall (also see Kirk and Dyrbye, 1957).

Stevens et al. (1976) were also able to demonstrate a decreased content of CSC in the intima and media of the atherosclerotic artery. This pattern of deposition in the arterial wall of these different mucopolysaccharides, along with the clinical evidence that has already been accumulated on the beneficial effects of CSC and CSA, is probably reason enough to limit CS administration to just CSC and CSA.

There is also evidence that mucopolysaccharide types in the blood vessel wall that are nonsulfated (like hyaluronic acid) will bind lipoproteins circulating in the blood, which would appear to support the development of atherosclerosis (Gero et al., 1961). Furthermore, when the content of these nonsulfated mucopolysaccharides in the arterial wall is documented to be low, the susceptibility to atherosclerosis in several animal species is also noted to be low (Engel, 1971).

As a practical point, then, products that are assayed as having mostly well-sulfated acid mucopolysaccharides like CSC and CSA should be the mucopolysaccharide supplements of choice unless further clinical research dictates that other less-sulfated or non-sulfated products have clearly positive clinical effects.

The effect of vitamin C in favorably affecting the levels of CSA in the arterial wall was examined by Verlangieri and Stevens (1979). Studying atherosclerosis in rabbits fed cholesterol, these researchers found that the vitamin C-supplemented animals had significantly higher levels of CSA in their aortas than in animals not receiving vitamin C.

EXHIBIT 41

Vitamin C supplementation shown to significantly increase levels of cholesterol-lowering CSA in arterial walls.

As CSA has been found to have anti-atherosclerosis properties, this vitamin C-facilitated accumulation of CSA in the arterial wall may be a significant mechanism by which vitamin C helps CSA exert these properties. This accumulation of CSA in the arterial wall may be at least partially explained by the work of Schwartz and Adamy (1976 and 1977).

Their experiments suggested that vitamin C inhibited an enzyme felt to break down CSA. Such an action would favor greater degrees of accumulation of CSA in the arterial wall.

Nakazawa and Murata (1975) also reported that roughly twice as many heart patients treated with CS versus those patients treated with placebo showed some improvement of the part of their electrocardiograms (ST-T segments) that often reveals diminished blood supply to the heart muscle. Nakazawa and Murata (1978) were later able to demonstrate one patient that underwent a dramatic normalization of the electrocardiogram from very striking abnormalities seen prior to treatment with CS.

In this particular patient, 3,000 mg of CS daily was given orally over the course of three years. The normalization of the electrocardiogram took a few months. Earlier, Nakazawa et al. (1969) were able to show that intravenous injections of CSC were able to improve the ST-T segments in about a third of the patients treated. The effects were observed anywhere from 30 to 180 minutes after CSC injection, persisting for several hours. Having both demonstrably positive acute and chronic effects on the electrocardiogram suggests that CS, especially the higher sulphur-containing CSC, is an especially good adjunctive agent to use in the treatment of chronic cardiac patients.

Even though Nakazawa and Murata (1978) found that CS has demonstrable cholesterol-lowering effects, the patient treated for three years just noted above had his chest pain and electrocardiographic abnormalities disappear even though the serum cholesterol levels "were not greatly altered." Most of their patients treated with CS had decreases in blood cholesterol ranging from 10% to 20%, while triglyceride levels were decreased by an average of 27%.

This again supports the conclusion that CS has multiple positive, although not always identical, effects on cardiac patients, and the lack of any significant side effects with these agents should warrant their routine use in cardiac patients. Whether one patient has, for example, a greater or lesser electrocardiographic or cholesterol response to CS therapy is not a good reason to limit its use for only selected patients.

The anticoagulant properties of CS, one of the properties noted above for CSA, are noteworthy as well. Today, most heart patients are given one or more antiplatelet drugs (Aljaroudi et al., 2005).

Platelets are the sticky elements of the blood that can initiate the process of forming a clot, or thrombus. Whenever a heart attack is caused by the sudden blocking off of a coronary artery, an abrupt clotting of the blood is nearly always involved.

Furthermore, after heart patients have had procedures such as balloon angioplasty with or without a mechanical stent to help keep the coronary artery open after the balloon inflation, some form of anticoagulant therapy is uniformly recommended.

CS is actually a member of a family of substances (acid mucopolysaccharides) that includes heparin, which is the most commonly prescribed intravenous agent for preventing the blood from clotting. In concert with the anti-atherosclerotic effects seen with CS, heparin has also been shown to have the ability to reduce the development of experimental cholesterol-induced atherosclerosis (Myasnikov, 1958).

This gives further general support to the concept that some form of acid mucopolysaccharide, probably CSC and/or CSA, should be routinely administered in patients with atherosclerosis.

Kirk (1959) published a study looking at the comparative anticoagulant abilities of different acid mucopolysaccharides. All substances tested had some anticoagulant ability. However, despite its superior anticoagulant properties, heparin is not as feasible a chronic therapeutic agent as CSC or CSA in humans since it must be given by needle, and since it is so effective in thinning the blood that bleeding complications can easily result.

Also, in addition to increasing the amount of time it takes for the blood to clot, CS has also been documented to actually lessen the size of a blood clot when clotting does occur. In rabbits, Nakazawa and Murata (1978) found that the weight of clots formed when CS was administered was less than the weight of clots formed when placebo was given.

Therefore, CS appears to be a very useful agent for the treatment and prevention of atherosclerosis and coronary heart disease. Furthermore, it appears that maintaining an optimal vitamin C status helps assure that the CS has an optimal sulfur content, which further appears to assure that the CS is optimally effective in its ability to combat the atherosclerotic process.

POLYUNSATURATED LECITHIN, ATHEROSCLEROSIS, CHOLESTEROL, AND VITAMIN C

Polyunsaturated lecithin, or polyunsaturated phosphatidylcholine (PPC), is another general term referring to a group of substances that directly impact the cholesterol metabolism in the arterial wall. Lecithin, or phosphatidylcholine, is a commonly used supplement today. The clinical and practical effects that the administration of PPC has on atherosclerosis will be cited, and the mechanisms by which PPC is believed to exert this effect will be discussed. The important interaction of vitamin C with PPC in the optimal expression of the anti-atherosclerotic properties of PPC will also be discussed.

One of the primary factors that determines whether a substance will ever become mobilized again after being deposited out of solution in the blood is its degree of solubility in water. The blood is most capable of transporting substances that are water-soluble. Many substances that dissolve very poorly in water, such as fats, can still be transported in the blood when they are in the proper chemical form to increase their water solubility.

Free cholesterol is the predominant form of cholesterol found in the lesions of both early and advanced atherosclerosis. This form of cholesterol is almost completely incapable of being directly dissolved in water. Because of this insolubility in water and the water-soluble nature of the blood, cholesterol deposited in a blood vessel without any subsequent alteration in its chemical composition may take months for its removal, if it gets removed at all. Such slow cholesterol removal and turnover can be expected to favor the process of accumulation in the blood vessel wall, with the progression of the atherosclerotic process rather than its reversal. Krumdieck and Butterworth (1974) note that only a limited number of mechanisms seem to exist for the removal of this type of cholesterol in the blood vessel wall:

- Transformation of the cholesterol into a more water-soluble derivative form,
- Alteration of the chemical nature of the circulating blood plasma such that unmodified cholesterol can be dissolved more easily into it, and
- Phagocytosis, or the actual ingestion of cholesterol crystals by special immune cells such as monocytes or macrophages.

The first mechanism is probably the best one to rely on most. Altering the solubility characteristics of the blood is not a very practical suggestion, although very appealing on a theoretical basis. Finally, phagocytosis will proceed spontaneously, but this mechanism probably also directly leads to early inner arterial wall thickening, as well as an ongoing stimulation to further inflammatory changes in the blood vessel wall.

As discussed earlier, anything that promotes an ongoing, chronic inflammatory response will also contribute to the progression of atherosclerosis. Finding a way to optimally stimulate and promote the redissolving of cholesterol out of the arterial wall is therefore very desirable. Furthermore, the presence of fewer resulting pockets of cholesterol crystals would stimulate less phagocytosis, which is desirable in lessening the further development of atherosclerosis.

How does one make the cholesterol in the blood vessel wall dissolve more readily back into the bloodstream? Simply, the cholesterol molecule must bind to another molecule that will result in an acceptable degree of water solubility.

A molecule containing an unsaturated fatty acid such as a PPC can transfer that fatty acid entity to the cholesterol molecule, resulting in what is known as cholesteryl ester, a substance with significantly more water solubility than free cholesterol. This cholesteryl ester is able to readily bind to HDL (Bielicki et al., 1995), which is then free to transport the cholesterol to the liver.

When PPC is the molecule that is contributing the fatty acid to the cholesterol molecule, an enzyme known as lecithin-cholesterol-acyl-transferase (LCAT) appears to be the primary catalyst promoting this transfer. The importance of this enzyme and the chemical reaction that it accelerates between PPC and the cholesterol in the blood vessel wall is revealed by the fact that individuals lacking this enzyme develop atherosclerosis at an early age (Norum et al., 1970).

Further indication of LCAT's likely importance in the prevention of atherosclerosis is that the activity level of this enzyme has been shown to be significantly reduced in patients with documented atherosclerotic heart disease relative to undiseased controls (Solajic-

Bozicevic et al., 1994), in patients who have survived heart attacks (Solajic-Bozicevic et al., 1991; Dobiasova, 1983), and in individuals with other established risk factors for developing atherosclerosis (Hovingh et al., 2005).

Santamarina-Fojo et al. (2000) have also noted that LCAT appears, by whatever mechanism, to increase the levels of HDL (the lipoprotein transporting cholesterol out of the blood vessel wall) and to lower the levels of LDL (the lipoprotein bringing cholesterol into the blood vessel wall). Rutenberg and Soloff (1971) had earlier suggested that LCAT seemed to react preferentially with HDL in helping to transfer a fatty acid from lecithin to free cholesterol.

It would appear that in the absence of this enzyme, cholesterol tends to make mostly a one-way trip into the blood vessel wall due to the lack of mechanisms to get cholesterol redissolved back into the bloodstream and subsequently transported, to the liver.

A saturated lecithin (SL) is much less effective than a PPC in promoting the synthesis of the desired final cholesterol product, a water-soluble cholesteryl ester. In a study on rats implanted with pellets of radioisotope-labeled cholesterol under the skin (subcutaneous), Adams and Morgan (1967) found that a highly unsaturated lecithin (PPC) was twice as effective as a saturated lecithin in increasing the rate of absorption of the cholesterol out of the implant and into the animal's body. Adams et al. (1967) were also able to demonstrate that the administration of a soybean-derived PPC was able to protect cholesterol-fed rabbits from the development of atherosclerosis. They also showed that a SL did not protect cholesterol-fed rabbits from the development of atherosclerosis.

There are multiple sources of lecithin in the supplement market. However, for the purposes of treating atherosclerosis it would appear that it is very important to take the polyunsaturated form of lecithin. Also, as a practical point, it would also appear that the soybean-derived lecithins are polyunsaturated and serve as good anti-atherosclerosis supplements.

In monkeys and hamsters Wilson et al. (1998) demonstrated that a soy lecithin-rich diet reduced total plasma cholesterol without reducing the HDL-bound, or "good" cholesterol. They also found that the early stages of atherosclerosis were significantly reduced in the hamsters as well.

In rabbits and rats Mastellone et al. (2000) found that the increased ingestion of soy lecithin had a cholesterol-lowering effect as well. Furthermore, they found that human endothelial cells incubated with soy lecithin were able to significantly rid themselves of the cholesterol they contained.

Polichetti et al. (1996) were also able to show that soy lecithin-rich diets in rats could also stimulate the liver's uptake of HDL-cholesterol. Polichetti et al. (2000) were also able to show significant increases in the amounts of cholesterol excreted into the bile via the liver in soy lecithin-fed rabbits. This indicates that soy lecithin not only helps the HDL get cholesterol out of the arterial wall, it also helps the HDL get rid of it into the liver and then into the bile, to be excreted in the intestine. These multiple positive effects that soy lecithin has on cholesterol metabolism appear to make it an optimal adjunctive therapy in the treatment of atherosclerosis.

So how does vitamin C interact with PPC in the effects that PPC has on cholesterol metabolism and the atherosclerotic process? Altman et al. (1980) were able to show that cholesterol-fed rabbits that would otherwise develop "extensive" atheromatous plaques developed no lesions at all when both vitamin C and lecithin therapy were given. The combination therapy was also superior in facilitating the regression of plaques that had already formed.

EXHIBIT 42

Combination of vitamin C and PPC shown to be much more effective at reversing plaques than either substance by itself.

However, use of either vitamin C or lecithin therapy singly, while showing a positive therapeutic effect in lessening the presence or hastening the resolution of plaques, was not able to completely prevent lesions or resolve existing lesions. Vitamin C alone, in the doses administered, was slightly less effective than lecithin alone in both prevention and regression of atherosclerosis in this experiment.

The positive anti-atherosclerotic interactions between the vitamin C therapy and the lecithin therapy seem to be quite significant. Vitamin C is known to help maintain the normal physical characteristics of the ground substance and basement membrane areas, making them substantially less receptive to the deposition of cholesterol from the blood. This one effect can help to explain how vitamin C and lecithin have better effects against atherosclerosis than either agent singly.

Additionally, by virtue of its antioxidant activity that provides so many other benefits in the body, vitamin C helps to prevent the reduction of LCAT activity by oxidizing factors (Chen and Loo, 1995). As with so many other enzymes, LCAT also appears to be subject to the negative effects of prooxidant factors, and vitamin C can nonspecifically help to protect LCAT from such stresses, a factor important in keeping LCAT levels optimal.

EXHIBIT 43

Vitamin C helps prevent destabilizing oxidation of LCAT activity.

Certainly, other positive interactions between vitamin C and lecithins are possible, and probably even likely, considering the widespread positive effects of vitamin C throughout the body. In any event, the interactions of lecithin and vitamin C help to underscore the importance of analyzing as completely as possible why a given medical condition develops, and then tailoring the therapies from as many intelligent directions as possible. Of course, any safe therapy known to be effective for a given medical condition should never be avoided simply because the mechanism of action is unknown or incompletely defined.

The contribution of excessive cholesterol to the development of atherosclerosis appears to be another risk factor that can be virtually eliminated in many patients if adequate daily vitamin C is taken. Through both the direct and indirect mechanisms discussed above, cholesterol has been demonstrated to be another risk factor for heart disease that requires vitamin C deficiency to exert its initial negative effects. Furthermore, ongoing vitamin C deficiency clearly accelerates the progression of atherosclerosis in the face of excessive cholesterol levels. In certain exceptional cases, vitamin C supplementation would only be able to lessen the degree to which cholesterol serves as a risk factor for atherosclerosis.

However, for most individuals without extraordinary toxin loads, adequate vitamin C dosing should normalize cholesterol levels and often render cholesterol of no significant consequence in the development of arterial blockages. The addition of nutrient substances such as CS and PPC only further help vitamin C negate the atherosclerotic effects of excessive cholesterol.

CHAPTER 6

Triglycerides and Vitamin C Deficiency

A triglyceride, like cholesterol, is another lipid (fat or fat-like substance) that has been linked to heart disease. An elevated level of triglycerides in the blood is an independent risk factor for having a greater chance of death by heart attack (Carlson and Bottiger, 1985). Hopkins et al. (2005) also found that the association between the total triglyceride level in the blood and premature familial coronary atherosclerosis "is strong, graded, and independent." Mennander et al. (2005) further found that an elevated triglyceride level is significant in predicting the need for repeat coronary artery bypass surgeries in the future. Kolovou et al. (2005) showed that patients with coronary artery atherosclerosis elevate their plasma triglyceride levels after a fatty meal higher than in patients without pre-existing atherosclerosis.

Vitamin C appears to positively affect triglyceride levels. Erden et al. (1985) found that 2,000 mg of vitamin C daily administered to a group of 50 volunteers over a two-month period decreased both the triglyceride and cholesterol levels, while increasing the HDL cholesterol fraction. However, not surprisingly, the dose of vitamin C appears to be critical in order to demonstrate this triglyceride-lowering effect. Bishop et al. (1985) did a similar study in diabetic patients, except that only 500 mg of vitamin C was given daily. Over a four-month period, no significant differences were seen in either the triglyceride or cholesterol levels.

EXHIBIT 44

Vitamin C dose-dependent studies show 2000 mg vitamin C daily lowers triglycerides where 500 mg does not.

Perhaps another reason for some of the mixed results seemingly reported in the literature on the effects of vitamin C on elevated triglyceride levels comes from the population of patients being studied.

Wahlberg and Walldius (1982) reported that 2,000 mg of vitamin C daily did not lower the serum triglycerides in the nine patients they treated. However, these patients all had an inherited disease characterized by elevated blood levels of triglycerides. Clearly, such a genetic disease can be expected to likely utilize different or additional mechanisms in the production of elevated triglycerides in the blood. Such a result cannot be used to summarily negate the conclusions of studies that report the ability of vitamin C to lower triglycerides in either normal patients or patients with other selected diseases.

Ness et al. (1996a) looked at the relationship of plasma vitamin C level to the serum triglyceride level.

They concluded that the plasma vitamin C level was negatively correlated with the triglyceride level, meaning the higher the vitamin C level, the lower the triglyceride level. They also concluded that their results were consistent with other published work that indicated that a high dietary intake of vitamin C not only lowered triglyceride levels, but also raised HDL cholesterol levels.

> **EXHIBIT 45**
>
> **High dietary intake of vitamin C not only lowers triglyceride levels but also raises HDL cholesterol levels.**

The effect of a combined antioxidant therapy on elevated serum triglyceride levels has also been studied. Hamilton et al. (2000) found that a combination of only 500 mg of vitamin C daily with a dosage of vitamin E was effective in lowering both triglyceride and total cholesterol levels. Using a similarly dosed combination of vitamins C and E, Babu et al. (2000) were also able to demonstrate the significant lowering of triglyceride levels that were elevated by the administration of tamoxifen. Tamoxifen is a non-steroidal antiestrogen drug used in the hormonal treatment of breast cancer. These authors suggested that addition of vitamins C and E to tamoxifen therapy was a superior form of treatment to tamoxifen alone.

In guinea pigs, Ha et al. (1990) also found that vitamin C had a relationship to the blood level of triglycerides. By feeding four groups of animals varying amounts of vitamin C, they were able to conclude that an inverse relationship existed between tissue levels of vitamin C and plasma levels of triglycerides. As in the studies already noted above, higher amounts of vitamin C were associated with lower amounts of triglycerides. These authors went so far as to suggest that vitamin C deficiency in guinea pigs may impair the metabolism, or breakdown, of triglycerides in the blood. Bobek et al. (1980), also studying guinea pigs, found that a "chronic borderline vitamin C deficiency" led to both elevated blood levels of triglycerides as well as the accumulation of triglycerides in the liver.

It would appear, then, that elevated levels of triglycerides in the blood are best supported by a state of vitamin C deficiency, along with inadequate dietary intake and supplementation of vitamin C. When an elevated level of triglycerides is present in the blood, exerting its effect as a risk factor for the development of atherosclerosis, a vitamin C deficiency can be expected to be present as well.

Undoubtedly, an excess presence of the fatty triglycerides works in concert with the vitamin C deficiency to both initiate and accelerate the development of atherosclerosis. It is also likely that any future clinical studies using substantially higher supplemented doses of vitamin C (for example, 5,000 to 15,000 mg daily) will consistently show a triglyceride-lowering effect from this supplementation.

CHAPTER 7
Lipoprotein(a) and Vitamin C Deficiency

Lipoproteins are any of a number of fat-protein complexes that serve to transport fat in the blood. As examples of this class of substances, commonly known lipoproteins are the high-density (HDL) and low-density lipoproteins (LDL), which are known primarily for their cholesterol transport functions. HDL transports cholesterol to the liver for metabolism and excretion, while LDL transports cholesterol to tissues other than the liver, including the arterial walls. Because of these transport characteristics, HDL-bound cholesterol is known as the "good" cholesterol and LDL-bound cholesterol is known as the "bad" cholesterol, at least in regard to the likelihood of developing atherosclerosis.

HDL is considered a good lipoprotein since a high blood level of it means there is a greater capacity for transporting more cholesterol out of the arterial walls to the liver for excretion into the intestine via the bile. Just the opposite is considered to be the case for

LDL, which is known to help bind cholesterol in the arterial wall.

Rath and Pauling (1990) looked in detail at another type of lipoprotein, known as lipoprotein(a),

EXHIBIT 46

Lipoprotein(a) assumes/shares some of vitamin C's many important functions when vitamin C deficient.

or Lp(a). They hypothesized that Lp(a) served as a surrogate, or substitute, for vitamin C. They noted that low vitamin C levels regularly resulted in a compensatory increase in Lp(a) plasma levels. They reported that Lp(a) was apparently being produced by the body in an attempt to compensate for inadequate vitamin C intake and the body's inability to synthesize vitamin C of its own. They felt that Lp(a) and vitamin C shared certain properties, including:

- the acceleration of wound healing (also see Brown and Goldstein, 1987)
- cell-repair mechanisms
- strengthening of the ground substance surrounding the cells in blood vessels
- preventing the degeneration of lipids, or fats.

In support of these assertions, Rath and Pauling also found that Lp(a) was found primarily in the plasma of animal species that could not synthesize vitamin C. Conversely, most of the animals that could synthesize their own vitamin C were found to have no detectable Lp(a) in their plasma.

Rath and Pauling (1990a) also noted that Lp(a) is a lipoprotein exceptionally adept in promoting atherosclerosis. von Eckardstein et al. (2001) found that Lp(a) emerged as an important independent coronary artery disease (atherosclerosis) risk factor, with the increased risk most pronounced when combined with the other risk factors of elevated LDL cholesterol, lowered HDL cholesterol, and hypertension. Furthermore, Stubbs et al. (1997) found that higher Lp(a) levels in unstable angina patients seemed to correlate with the patients most likely to proceed to a significant cardiac complication, such as blockage of the artery and heart attack.

> **EXHIBIT 47**
>
> **High levels of Lipoprotein(a) – thought to be an indicator of vitamin C deficiency – contributes to atherosclerosis.**

Rath and Pauling basically felt that an increased Lp(a) level in the body was a compensatory mechanism of the body for vitamin C deficiency. When the Lp(a) levels were high enough for a long enough period of time, this compensatory mechanism essentially "overcompensated," and the same actions of Lp(a) that initially protected the blood vessels became a major player in damaging them.

One of the components of Lp(a), apoprotein(a) [apo(a)], was felt by Rath and Pauling to be an effective antioxidant, which perhaps helps to explain why Lp(a) could serve to help substitute for vitamin C in the body. However, unlike vitamin C, a prolonged excessive presence of Lp(a) results in its excessive deposition in the arterial wall. This directly promotes the development of atherosclerosis (Rath et al., 1989), and effectively negates the clinical benefit of any antioxidant effects.

Minimal deposition of Lp(a) in the blood vessel wall, although still contributing to the original development of atherosclerosis, might play a greater role early on in strengthening the blood vessel wall compromised by vitamin C deficiency. Continued, unchecked deposition would clearly become far more detrimental than helpful to blood vessel health.

Rath and Pauling (1991) also suggested that vitamin C deficiency increases plasma concentrations of Lp(a) and fibrinogen because of the abilities of these two substances to combat bleeding complications. Fibrinogen is a substance that is known to increase the clotting ability of the blood, converting into fibrin after the clotting process is initiated. The fibrin makes up the bulk of the blood clot.

Even though Lp(a) and fibrinogen/fibrin complexes both end up as significant components of the mature atherosclerotic plaque, their early appearance in the development of atherosclerosis may be necessary to prevent the early, potentially fatal, bleeding complications of substantial vitamin C deficiency.

Niendorf et al. (1990) were able to demonstrate Lp(a) deposition in the arterial wall and find that its presence correlated with the extent of atherosclerotic lesion development in the coronary arteries and the aorta. Cushing et al. (1989) were able to show that Lp(a) accumulation also appeared to be significant in the development of atherosclerosis in coronary artery bypass vein grafts. A vein graft lacks the external support in the blood vessel wall found in an artery, and this lack may also contribute to the "need" for Lp(a) to exert its initial protective effect in the absence of adequate vitamin C.

As noted earlier, vitamin C deficiency promptly and directly results in the breaking down of the linkages (polymerization) of the glycoprotein molecules in the basement membrane supporting the endothelial cells lining the arteries. This was already noted to change the consistency of the basement membrane from being jelly-like to being more watery and runny (Gersh and Catchpole, 1949; Pirani and Catchpole, 1951). Just as with cholesterol, this vitamin C deficiency-induced defect in the integrity of the basement membrane allows Lp(a) and other blood fats, such as cholesterol, to infiltrate this weakened intimal area and start the process of atherosclerosis.

Rath and Pauling (1990) suggest an additional mechanism by which vitamin C can lessen the ability of Lp(a) to promote atherosclerosis. Fibrin, a common component in the maturing plaque as well as at a site of arterial injury (which often initiates atherosclerosis), helps to bind Lp(a) to the plaque. Rath and Pauling (1991a) provided evidence that a protein component of Lp(a) is very prone to sticking to other tissues.

Rath and Pauling (1990) also suggested that since this stickiness involves the Lp(a) sticking to sites containing lysine (an amino acid), which is found in the fibrin component of the plaque, vitamin C may alter the lysine chemically so that it will no longer bind Lp(a). Scanu et al. (1994) later demonstrated the presence and importance of this lysine binding site in the binding of Lp(a) to lysine in humans. This modification of lysine by vitamin C would likely significantly diminish the contribution of Lp(a) to growing sites of atherosclerosis, since its ability to stick to those sites would be lessened.

Keeping the above reasoning in mind, Pauling (1994) asserted that since binding sites containing lysine could attach Lp(a) to the arterial wall, then taking more lysine in supplemental form would competitively bind to Lp(a) before it had a chance to bind to arterial wall lysine. Pauling said this would not only decrease Lp(a) binding to the arterial wall, it might even work to dislodge Lp(a) already bound if enough lysine were taken, thereby playing a significant role in lessening the bulk of the plaque and reversing atherosclerosis.

Boonmark et al. (1997) were able to demonstrate in mice that the lysine binding site in Lp(a) was very important in the development of atherosclerosis. They were able to demonstrate that mice with specific mutations that destroyed this lysine binding site greatly reduced the ability of the Lp(a) to bind lysine. And most significantly, they were able to demonstrate that mice with such mutations were less likely to develop atherosclerosis, further indicating the likely importance of lysine's ability to further bind more Lp(a) and increase the bulk of the arterial lesion.

In three case reports, (Pauling, 1991; Pauling, 1993; McBeath and Pauling, 1993) Pauling repeatedly observed the dramatic reduction of anginal (heart-related) chest pains with a regimen of lysine and vitamin C. Interestingly, Pauling also noted that the response of these three patients had been rapid, within two to four weeks of initiating the treatment. The doses of vitamin C and lysine ranged from 3,000 mg to 6,000 mg of each daily. It is also notewor-thy that two of the patients had ad-vanced coronary artery disease, having already had coronary by-pass surgeries. However, the other one had no blockages in the major

EXHIBIT 48

Large daily doses of vitamin C and comparable doses of lysine reduce anginal chest pains.

arteries on angiography, indicating either small vessel disease or coronary artery spasm, or both. Neverthe-less, Pauling's regimen was equally effective in reduc-ing anginal chest pains in all three patients.

There is at least one good reason for the uniform-ly good response that Pauling observed in his three cardiac patients placed on vitamin C and lysine.

Anginal chest pain typically occurs when there is enough of a restriction of blood flow to an area of the heart muscle. Coronary (heart) artery blood flow is affected both by fixed arterial blockages and by the general caliber of the blood vessel. Variable amounts of muscular contraction in the wall of the artery (spasm or vasomotor tone) can restrict blood flow enough to cause angina even without fixed blockages present.

EXHIBIT 49

Vitamin C able to restore impaired blood flow through heart and small blood vessels.

This spasm of the blood vessel can also superimpose itself at times on a fixed blockage and cause an im-mediate significant compromise of the blood flow as well. Kaufmann et al. (2000) showed that vitamin C was able to restore the impaired blood flow throughout the heart and the small blood vessels (microcirculation) typically seen in smokers. This strongly implies that the clinical entity known as coronary artery spasm responds very well to the administration of vitamin C. Although long-term treatment with Pauling's regimen may well also end up showing regression of atherosclerotic lesions, the quick symptomatic response that he found in his three case reports was probably due to a relaxation of muscle tone in the coronary arteries, with resulting improved blood flow to the heart muscle.

Rath (1992) suggested the addition of proline (another amino acid) supplementation to further augment the likely antiatherosclerosis effects of vitamin C and lysine. Lysine is known to competitively inhibit the binding of Lp(a) to fibrinogen, fibrin, and fibrin-related products, which are typical components of the developing atherosclerotic plaque. Similarly, proline appears to also play an important role in binding Lp(a) to plaque. Trieu et al. (1991) showed that proline and its related compound hydroxyproline bind to Lp(a). Collagen, which is rich in proline compounds, comprises a significant portion of the maturing, fibrous plaques. The addition of proline supplementation to a patient's regimen should be expected to bind increased amounts of Lp(a) before that Lp(a) has the chance to bind the proline-rich compounds in the developing atherosclerotic plaque, thereby preventing the Lp(a) from sticking to the plaque and increasing its bulk.

As with the reasoning already presented for the administration of lysine as an antiatherosclerotic agent, proline supplementation should also be expected to lessen the amount of Lp(a) that would stick to any other proline-rich constituents in the blood vessel wall. This should also be expected to decrease the development and/or progression of atherosclerosis. As with lysine, it is also suggested that high enough doses of proline could eventually displace some Lp(a) already bound to a developing plaque, thereby releasing the Lp(a) into the bloodstream, debulking the plaque, and eventually resulting in objective regression of the atherosclerotic narrowing.

Most chemical bonds have some practical level of dynamic equilibrium in which those bonds are continuing to form and break, such as is seen with different salts in solution. When enough of another substance is present that will also bond with a given chemical site, some of it will eventually physically displace some of what was already bound there first through this ongoing mechanism of bond breaking and new bond formation. By such a mechanism, lysine and proline could actually lessen the content of Lp(a) in a blood vessel wall or atherosclerotic lesion over time. Rath (1992) asserted that human atherosclerotic lesions are primarily composed of Lp(a), so having the ability to displace this substance specifically from plaque could play an enormous role in reversing even advanced atherosclerotic lesions.

By administering vitamin C, lysine, and proline, along with niacin, guar gum, and the ayurvedic herb gum guggulu, Katz (1996) was able to achieve some very impressive results in a 62 year-old female heart patient. Each of the above agents was documented individually to significantly lower this patient's Lp(a) level. Repeat angiography of this patient's heart arteries revealed very significant improvements during the approximately 19-month treatment period between the two studies. A narrowing of 75% in the right coronary was reduced to a 40% narrowing. Also, other narrowings of approximately 50% were no longer seen. Although this is a positive result in only one patient, the response was a very dramatic one, and the lowering of the Lp(a) level with each therapeutic agent given would seem to indicate that bringing this particular laboratory test into the normal range is very critical in treating such cardiac patients.

As with the other risk factors, it would appear that vitamin C deficiency "sets the stage" for optimizing the abilities of Lp(a) to initiate and promote the development of atherosclerosis.

Vitamin C deficiency promptly alters the chemical composition and consistency of the basement membrane supporting the endothelial cells lining the inner wall of the artery. As discussed earlier with cholesterol, this change in the nature of the basement membrane also makes it easier for Lp(a) and other blood fats to start depositing there.

That same vitamin C deficiency also simultaneously helps to elevate the circulating levels of Lp(a), which presumably initially appears to help compensate for the vitamin C deficiency. Before too long, however, excess amounts of Lp(a) become deposited in the weakened arterial walls, and atherosclerosis is well underway. Administration of adequate amounts of vitamin C not only brings the levels of Lp(a) down, it also appears that such dosages lessen the likelihood that any Lp(a) remaining in circulation will get deposited.

The supplementation of the amino acids lysine and proline would also appear to contribute to the slowing, and possibly reversal, of the atherosclerotic process. As discussed in the cholesterol risk factor section, the chances of atherosclerosis reversibility with these measures will largely hinge on whether the patient's daily toxin exposure can be adequately neutralized with enough daily vitamin C. Such toxin sources as root canal-treated teeth and other infected teeth can be expected to largely block the ability of vitamin C and other supplements to reverse atheroslerosis, even if some clinical benefit can be observed.

CHAPTER 8
Diabetes and Vitamin C Deficiency

Diabetes is a well-established risk factor for atherosclerosis and coronary heart disease (Dahl-Jorgensen et al., 2005; Haffner, 2005). Diabetes, or more precisely, diabetes mellitus, is a chronic disease in which the metabolism of carbohydrate, protein, and fat is impaired due to the inadequate production of insulin or due to resistance of the target tissues to the effects of insulin. As with the other risk factors, diabetes rarely exists as the sole risk factor for heart disease in a given patient. Very commonly, hypertension and lipid disorders (such as elevated Lp(a) and elevated cholesterol) coexist with diabetes.

Diabetes is a disease in which there are significantly increased levels of oxidative stress. Such increased oxidative stress can result from increased free radical production and/or reduced antioxidant defenses (Hunt et al., 1992; Gupta and Chari, 2005). Indeed, many of the complications of diabetes are felt to be secondary to this increased oxidative stress (Wolff et al., 1991; Baynes, 1991). Sato et al. (1979) were able to show that some of the blood vessel complications commonly seen in diabetes occur when there is evidence of increased oxidative stress in the blood.

In addition to any other mechanisms by which vitamin C levels can be reduced in diabetes, the increased production of free radicals will always reliably utilize vitamin C. Such utilization will result in lower levels of vitamin C in the blood and the tissues. Multiple studies have shown that diabetics have reduced plasma levels of vitamin C (Ginter et al., 1978; Som et al., 1981; Stankova et al., 1984; Mooradian and Morley, 1987; Simon, 1992).

EXHIBIT 50

Multiple studies show that diabetics have depressed, scurvy-like plasma levels of vitamin C.

Price et al. (1996) advanced the proposition that the elevated glucose level (hyperglycemia) seen in diabetes can directly induce a state of latent scurvy, or advanced vitamin C deficiency. This latent scurvy was felt to be characterized by a reversible form of atherosclerosis, depending upon the availability of vitamin C.

One likely, and perhaps primary, mechanism by which diabetes promotes atherosclerosis is by its ability to induce and maintain significantly low levels of vitamin C. Once a condition exists that can keep the vitamin C levels low enough in the body, the stage is set for virtually all of the other mechanisms already discussed to start and advance the development of atherosclerosis.

Hyperglycemia is probably the single most characteristic blood finding in diabetes. Although nearly all chronic medical diseases are associated with decreased vitamin C levels in the body due to increased demands for, and increased consumption of, vitamin C by the disease process itself, diabetes has some additional mechanisms depleting the body's tissue levels of vitamin C.

It has been well-established that glucose competes with vitamin C for uptake into the cell and mitochondria (Bigley et al., 1983; Kapeghian and Verlangieri, 1984; Khatami et al., 1986; Sagun et al., 2005; Wilson, 2005). Therefore, the sicker diabetic patients with the higher, more poorly controlled blood glucose levels will be expected to have

> **EXHIBIT 51**
> Vitamin C competes with glucose for uptake in the cells and mitochondria (the cells energy plant).

lower levels of vitamin C in their cells than nondiabetics or diabetics with less elevated blood glucose levels. Greater amounts of glucose will always result in lower cellular levels of vitamin C due to this direct competition between glucose and vitamin C for transport into the cell.

Insulin, the pancreatic hormone needed to metabolize glucose and maintain normal levels of it in the blood, is typically deficient in patients with diabetes. Hyperglycemia is usually the result of such an insulin deficiency in the body. Cunningham (1998) noted that insulin promotes the cellular uptake of vitamin C as well as the cellular uptake of glucose. Sherry and Ralli (1948) had earlier noted that an injection of insulin resulted in a fall in the plasma levels of vitamin C and a rise in the white blood cell and platelet levels of vita-

EXHIBIT 52

Insulin, usually deficient in diabetics, aids transport of vitamin C into the cells throughout the body.

min C. One straightforward reason for this observation is simply that the insulin takes the vitamin C out of the blood and pushes it into the white blood cells and platelets.

Vitamin C is very similar in chemical structure to glucose, helping to explain why insulin aids the cellular uptake of both glucose and vitamin C. Therefore, the natural state of diabetes, with elevated blood levels of glucose and lowered blood levels of insulin, has two separate factors that operate to help assure a cellular deficiency of vitamin C.

Mann (1974), with some of the above interactions in mind, hypothesized that the role of insulin in transporting vitamin C into certain tissues could explain some of the clinical findings in diabetes, a disease characterized by impaired insulin function.

Mann (1974) asserted that certain insulin-sensitive tissues in diabetics lacked vitamin C. He considered this lack of vitamin C to produce a "local scurvy," with the poor local collagen formation that one would then anticipate. He felt that one of the most susceptible tissues to this focal depletion of vitamin C is the vascular wall. He also felt that the competition between vitamin C and glucose for the same transport mechanism into the cell would allow a large enough dose of vitamin C to prevail in putting sufficient amounts of vitamin C inside the cells.

Furthermore, he also asserted that a large intake of vitamin C with "adequate insulin" would further assure delivery of the vitamin C into the cells, thereby preventing atherosclerotic lesions.

In addition to the effects that hyperglycemia has on lowering the cellular levels of vitamin C, hyperglycemia also works to lower vitamin C levels in the blood. Although the general metabolism of the diabetic state works to consume more vitamin C just like most other chronic degenerative diseases, the hyperglycemia seen with diabetes also has an effect on the kidneys that tends to waste increased amounts of vitamin C through the urine. Will and Byers (1996) have noted that hyperglycemia works to decrease the ability of the natural filters in the kidney to reabsorb the vitamin C that gets presented to it. This results in more vitamin C being excreted in the urine and less vitamin C being returned to the blood.

> **EXHIBIT 53**
>
> **High blood sugar forces the kidneys to remove and discard valuable vitamin C from the blood.**

Fisher et al. (1991) were able to show that high glucose levels can also inhibit some important functions of vitamin C. In cultured fibroblasts, vitamin C increased the production of collagen and proteoglycan content in the culture medium. However, in the presence of a high concentration of glucose, the stimulation of collagen and proteoglycan production by fibroblasts was impaired. Furthermore, these researchers found that insulin could block the inhibitory action that

> **EXHIBIT 54**
>
> **Excess blood glucose inhibits important functions of vitamin C.**

glucose excess exerted on this collagen production, although they were unable to offer a clear explanation for these observations. However, they were able to say that the inhibitory effect of glucose excess on the vitamin C-stimulated production of collagen by fibroblasts was not due to the inhibition of vitamin C uptake by the fibroblasts. The conclusion to be reached from this study is that hyperglycemia can suppress one of the primary functions of vitamin C, collagen synthesis. Insulin, on the other hand, has the positive effect of promoting this activity of vitamin C by somehow blocking the effect of hyperglycemia.

In any event, the high blood glucose and low blood insulin usually seen in diabetics both work to help impair vitamin C-mediated collagen synthesis. This again makes a vital vitamin C-related function something of a "final common pathway" for the expression of the negative effects that diabetes has on the development of atherosclerosis. Simply, the less readily collagen can be synthesized by the fibroblasts in the blood vessel wall, the more readily those blood vessels will be primed for the continued development of atherosclerosis.

EXHIBIT 55

High blood glucose depletes vitamin C from monocytes – white blood cells that gather at sites of inflammation and infection.

Chen et al. (1983) demonstrated that hyperglycemia was also especially effective in depleting the vitamin C content in monocytes. Monocytes are the white blood cells that often show up at sites of inflammation and infection, and proceed to ingest foreign material (phagocytosis). Depleting these cells of vitamin C directly impairs the defensive abilities of the immune system. This is likely a primary reason for the presence of the severe and rapidly developing blood vessel disease often seen in poorly controlled diabetic patients.

Indeed, relative to nondiabetics with atherosclerosis, the atherosclerotic plaques in diabetics are larger, with a greater fat (lipid) content, and more widespread in the blood vessels (Burke et al., 2001).

Platelets, the sticky elements in the blood that often directly affect the initiation of a blood clot, also have decreased levels of vitamin C in diabetic patients. Vitamin E, another very important antioxidant in the body, is also significantly depleted in the platelets of diabetic patients (Karpen et al., 1984). Sarji et al. (1979) published evidence that indicated greater amounts of vitamin C in platelets directly correlated to a lessened tendency to aggregate, or initiate the focus for a blood clot.

EXHIBIT 56
Diabetics develop larger atherosclerotic plaques with greater fat content.

Furthermore, they showed that this effect was not only demonstrable in a test tube, but also readily demonstrable in human subjects. They found that the oral administration of 2,000 mg of vitamin C daily in "normal non-smoking males" resulted in a "marked inhibition" of platelets sticking together. Blood clotting is an integral part of the progression of the small vessel disease (angiopathy) seen in diabetics, and this anti-platelet sticking effect of vitamin C is typically less in evidence in the diabetic. This represents one more vitamin C deficiency-mediated role for the progression of vascular disease seen in diabetics.

Vitamin C also directly relates to fibrinolytic activity, or the ability to dissolve clots that have already been formed. Bordia et al. (1978) showed that this clot-busting activity in the blood remains high as long as the blood level of vitamin C remains high. With this effect and the effect noted above on platelets, it would appear that the low levels

EXHIBIT 57

Vitamin C has the ability to help dissolve dangerous blood clots after they have already been formed.

of vitamin C seen in diabetes can make blood clots likelier to form and less likely to dissolve. Will et al. (1999) were able to show that the average vitamin C levels in the blood were "significantly lower" in persons with newly diagnosed diabetes than in nondiabetics. Clinically supporting the above observations, Spittle (1973 and 1974) was able to demonstrate that vitamin C administration has a powerful protective effect against unwanted blood clotting.

Vitamin C also appears to play an essential role in regulating the release of insulin from the cells that produce it in the pancreas (Dou et al., 1997), demonstrating further the involved interplay between these two substances. Also, Banerjee and Ghosh (1947) noted that scurvy-stricken guinea pigs do not metabolize glucose as effectively as normal guinea pigs.

EXHIBIT 58

Vitamin C plays an essential role in regulating the release of insulin by the pancreas.

In explanation of this abnormal glucose metabolism, they also demonstrated that the actual insulin content in the pancreas of such vitamin C-deprived animals was only about 25% of that found in the pancreas of normal animals. They were also able to conclude that the decreased insulin content of the pancreas in scurvy was primarily due to the lack of vitamin C and not due to a generally poor nutritional status.

Banerjee (1943) had already earlier noted that guinea pigs with scurvy had much lower levels of insulin in the pancreas than found in normal animals. Furthermore, he noted that the normal metabolism of glucose was restored after the administration of vitamin C.

Banerjee (1944) later was able to look at the pancreas of guinea pigs microscopically, finding that the number of insulin-producing cells in the pancreas was increased even though the total content of insulin in the pancreas was decreased. All of this data would seem to indicate that vitamin C has an important role in the synthesis of insulin (Kodama et al., 1993) in addition to its role in the release of insulin already synthesized and stored in the pancreas.

Therapeutically speaking, the evidence indicates that the regular administration of vitamin C is extremely important for the optimal treatment of diabetes. Kodama et al. (1993) found that diabetic patients showed superior clinical improvement when an infusion of vitamin C was combined with the insulin injections.

The very fact that vitamin C is so critical in the optimal management of diabetes again underscores the fact that diabetes and vitamin C deficiency are two closely interrelated conditions. In guinea pigs, the condition of scurvy reliably induces a state of pre-diabetes, with diminished insulin formation and an easy propensity to develop elevated blood glucose levels (Banerjee and Bandyopadhyay, 1963).

Furthermore, such states of scurvy-induced pre-diabetes are completely reversible by the administration of vitamin C. In many ways, diabetes would appear to be a disease that is an especially exaggerated picture of the consequences of a significant, protracted deficiency of vitamin C, particularly inside the cells.

Individuals with diabetes are also much more

EXHIBIT 59

Diabetics much more likely to have advanced periodontal disease.

likely to have advanced periodontal disease than nondiabetics (Belting et al., 1964). As already noted in the section above on inflammation as a risk factor for atherosclerosis, periodontal disease is associated with an increased risk of heart attack. Aleo (1981) proposed that vitamin C deficiency further contributes to the development of periodontal disease in diabetics through a number of different mechanisms. This likely represents yet one more way by which diabetes promotes atherosclerosis with the help of a vitamin C deficiency.

To recap, diabetes appears to exert much, if not most, of its negative impact on the body by virtue of the chronic deficiency of vitamin C in both the tissues and the blood seen with this disease.

The local deficit of vitamin C in the blood vessel wall induced by diabetes can easily initiate the atherosclerotic process. After this initial damage to the blood vessel wall, other risk factors such as inflammation and elevated blood fats like cholesterol and Lp(a) can more easily make their contributions to plaque development.

Finally, the unique interrelationship between insulin and vitamin C also offers strong evidence that diabetes is not just another disease that exerts its negative effect by metabolizing huge amounts of vitamin C. Indeed, the chronic diabetic state is both the result of vitamin C deficiency and a very strong contributor to a continuing state of significant vitamin C deficiency, even if the reason for the initial development of the diabetes is known and is not directly related to vitamin C deficiency.

CHAPTER 9
Age, Genetics, Gender, and Vitamin C Deficiency

AGE AND VITAMIN C

Increasing age is also associated with an increasing incidence of atherosclerosis and heart attack. In fact, Allison and Wright (2005) have provided evidence that age is the predominant risk factor for coronary artery calcification, later discussed as an independent risk factor for premature coronary heart disease.

While undoubtedly a multifaceted risk factor, increasing age also correlates with decreasing blood and tissue levels of vitamin C. In addition to the poor nutrition of many elderly people, Wilson et al. (1973) pointed out that older patients often endure a "wide variety of stressful states," including illnesses of variable degrees of severity. They attributed the low vitamin C levels in the white blood cells and platelets of this geriatric population to be more likely the result of these factors than just a poor dietary intake of vitamin C.

Regardless, the bottom line for many older people is that their blood and tissue vitamin C levels are lower than younger people. This would be at least one good reason why older patients have more heart disease than younger patients. Furthermore, Licastro et al. (2005) have noted that the older an individual is, the more likely that person is to have endured the presence of chronic systemic inflammation, which itself is a very significant risk factor for atherosclerosis.

However, this is not to say that vitamin C supplementation will not correct the vitamin C depletions often seen in the elderly. Newton et al. (1985) noted that the low vitamin C levels seen in both the blood and the white blood cells of the institutionalized and chronically sick elderly were correctable.

Schorah et al. (1979) showed that elderly long-stay inpatients with low levels of vitamin C in the blood and white blood cells responded well clinically to the administration of 1,000 mg of vitamin C daily. However, many elderly individuals never get their depleted vitamin C levels addressed, and this would appear to be one of the significant reasons why atherosclerosis generally worsens with increasing age.

GENETICS AND VITAMIN C

A positive family history of heart disease is considered by many to be an independent risk factor for coronary heart disease (Jorde and Williams, 1988).

However, genetic and environmental influences on the risk of developing heart disease can be difficult to distinguish apart from each other.

Although there do exist families that share definite genetic traits that predispose to heart disease (Austin et al., 1990), most families also share important dietary factors. These factors can predispose to heart disease directly, and they can also lead to other established risk factors for heart disease, such as hypertension, diabetes, obesity, and elevated lipids (cholesterol, triglycerides, and lipoproteins).

And as shared dietary and environmental influences in families lead to these other established risk factors, a shared vitamin C deficiency can occur as well, as discussed with the individual risk factors.

GENDER AND VITAMIN C

It is well known that more coronary artery disease and atherosclerosis develops in males than females. Tatsukawa et al. (2004) demonstrated that the male sex is an independent risk factor for atherosclerosis. Although there are a number of differences between men and women that could help account for this difference, vitamin C deficiency again appears as a significant, if not primary reason, for this observed difference.

Dodds (1969) studied the importance of gender as a factor in the blood levels of vitamin C. She noted that boys and girls between 4 and 12 years of age demonstrated little difference in their blood levels of vitamin C. However, she noted that males between

13 and 20 years of age began to show lower levels of vitamin C in the blood in the face of equivalent intakes of vitamin C. Finally, she found that this difference in blood vitamin C levels persisted between males and females aged 20 years and older. Earlier, Morgan et al. (1955) found that not only did men over 50 years of age have lower blood levels of vitamin C than comparably aged women, they also noted that wom-

EXHIBIT 60

Men have significantly lower vitamin C levels than comparably aged women.

en often had higher levels of vitamin C than men in spite of higher intakes of vitamin C by those men.

Furthermore, the magnitude of the difference in vitamin C levels discovered by Morgan et al. were quite significant. In the men and women over 50 years of age, they found that the women had an average blood vitamin C level of 1.07 mg per 100 ml, while the average level in the men was 0.83 mg per 100 ml. This means that on the basis of gender alone, the women had levels of vitamin C in their blood almost 30% greater than found in the men.

Franz et al. (1956), in studying nursing students and medical students, found comparable differences in the average blood vitamin C levels, even in these much younger individuals. The women in this younger group had vitamin C levels nearly 40% greater than found in the men.

Even when both groups received equal amounts of vitamin C supplementation, with significant rises seen in the blood levels of vitamin C, the women still maintained vitamin C levels more than 20% greater than found in the men.

Based on all of the mechanisms already discussed on the importance of vitamin C deficiency to the development and progression of atherosclerosis, it would appear that the greater vitamin C deficiency found in men is reason enough for men to have more of this disease than women of the same age.

Morgan et al. also noted that as men and women aged further, there was a tendency for the blood levels of vitamin C to show a convergence, with a lessening of the difference. Clinically, older patients of either sex with established coronary heart disease and atherosclerosis tend to evolve comparably, which meshes well with this convergence of blood vitamin C levels.

However, men should not feel that they are doomed to having a risk factor that they are unable to eliminate or largely negate. In the test tube, where conditions could be more rigidly controlled than in the body, Loh et al. (1974) found that there was no difference between men and women in the ability of their white blood cells to take up vitamin C from the plasma. It seems likely that optimal daily dosing of vitamin C by men would probably largely neutralize their increased risk of atherosclerosis relative to women.

However, the dosing of vitamin C may end up needing to be in the 6,000 to 12,000 mg per day for most men to block the effects of sex as a risk factor. Furthermore, for very large men who are very active physically, this proposed amount might need to be further increased substantially.

CHAPTER 10
Refined Sugar and Vitamin C Deficiency

The consumption of refined sugar in the diet is recognized to be an independent risk factor for the development of cardiovascular disease (Steward et al., 1995), although it is little addressed as a risk factor in the current medical and cardiological scientific literature and textbooks.

The statistical evidence certainly supports the position that sugar be considered a very significant risk factor for heart disease. At the very least, there is a clear correlation between increased refined sugar consumption and heart disease, even if it cannot be definitely asserted that this correlation is the equivalent of a cause-and-effect relationship.

However, this burden of demonstrating cause-and-effect after establishing a clear statistical correlation between risk factor and heart disease is shared by a number of the other cardiac risk factors being discussed.

The term "refined sugar" will be used in this section to refer primarily to the sucrose that is refined and concentrated from beets and sugar cane. However, corn-derived sugar will also have to be added to this category.

Fructose, as is ingested with the consumption of different fruits, may not have the same impact as the other sugars noted above, as the glucose rise in the blood after ingesting fructose is much less pronounced than with the other sugars.

Nevertheless, moderation is important in the ingestion of all purified sugars that ultimately release glucose into the bloodstream. As we shall see, it appears that both the amount of glucose in the blood and the rate of its rise in concentration are factors that directly relate to the development of atherosclerosis and coronary heart disease.

Refined sugar consumption has skyrocketed over the last century, both in the United States and across the world. Even the poorer countries maintain high consumption levels of the inexpensive refined sugars. Not much more than a century ago, the average amount of sugar consumed annually in the United States was about ten pounds per person. By 1980 this figure was up to about 125 pounds per person annually. And by 1994 the amount was almost a full 150 pounds (Yudkin, 1972; Dufty, 1975; Steward et al., 1995).

As it turns out, heart disease used to be a relatively rarity as a cause of death. Toward the end of the 1800s and into the early 1900s death by heart attack was uncommon. Although one may argue that many people died from other causes earlier in life before having the "chance" to die from heart disease, heart attacks appear to have increased in incidence in almost direct proportion to the incredible escalation of sugar consumption between 1900 and 2000.

EXHIBIT 61

Heart attacks have escalated in direct proportion with the increase in refined sugar consumption.

Heart attacks and heart-related diseases have gone from almost inconsequential in number at the turn of the century to now eventually claiming the lives of approximately half the population in the United States.

As mentioned in the earlier section on diabetes as a risk factor for atherosclerosis and heart disease, it has been clearly established that glucose, as well as a sizeable number of related sugars, directly competes with vitamin C for the same transport mechanism into the cells of the body (Mann and Newton, 1975; Bigley et al., 1983; Kapeghian and Verlangieri, 1984; Khatami et al., 1986).

Therefore, it would appear that the more glucose and other sugars are available in the blood, the less vitamin C will accumulate inside the cells of the body. Furthermore, when considering that sugar and vitamin C compete for the same transport

EXHIBIT 62

Sugars compete for the same transport mechanism for entrance in to the body's cells.

mechanism into the cell, it is perfectly logical to conclude that when glucose "spikes" rapidly into the blood, more glucose will be immediately transported inside the cells than vitamin C, which is not increasing in concentration in the blood at the same time.

On the other hand, when vitamin C levels are high and glucose is continuously but very slowly released into the blood, the concentration of glucose remains low at any one time, and vitamin C transport into the cells can predominate over the competing, but less concentrated, levels of glucose.

This suppression of vitamin C transport into the cells of the body by an excess presence of sugar in the blood would appear to be at least one significant mechanism by which sugar can stimulate the development of atherosclerosis and heart disease.

As discussed earlier, a deficiency of vitamin C in the lining cells inside the arteries is likely the first and primary change leading to atherosclerosis. Excess sugar would be expected to lower the levels of vitamin C in these endothelial cells of the arteries as well as everywhere else the sugar and vitamin C directly compete for entry into the cells.

It would appear that refined sugars are especially adept at rapidly elevating glucose levels in the bloodstream, which is likely a primary reason that such sugars are so effective in preventing optimal vitamin C entry into the cells, as noted above.

This ability to spike glucose into the bloodstream is reflected in the glycemic index of a food or nutrient substance (Foster-Powell and Miller, 1995). High glycemic index foods cause a quick rush of glucose into the blood, and low glycemic index foods release glucose into the blood much more gradually.

When considering the negatives of refined sugars in the diet, one should also be aware of the glycemic index ratings of all the foods regularly eaten. Eating certain high glycemic index foods frequently and in substantial amounts can result in a significant glucose spiking into the bloodstream, with the same effect of suppressing vitamin C entry into the cells as would be seen in the eating of refined sugars.

Not surprisingly, an increased consumption of high glycemic index foods has also been correlated with an increased incidence of coronary heart disease (Morris and Zemel, 1999; Liu et al., 2000; Ford and Liu, 2001). Also, a diet high in these same foods has also been correlated with a lower level of HDL cholesterol (Ford and Liu, 2001). Discussed more below, a lower HDL cholesterol level correlates both with increased heart disease and a higher consumption of sugars such as sucrose.

Excess consumption of refined sugar can also lead to and interact with other established risk factors for atherosclerosis and coronary heart disease. Long-term heavy sugar intake can be one factor in developing diabetes. Also, heavy sugar intake can lead to obesity, another known risk factor to be discussed later. Perhaps less well recognized is the documented ability of high sugar intake to directly interfere with the metabolism of cholesterol and blood fats, including triglycerides.

A fairly clear relationship between cholesterol and sucrose intake has been established. Generally, the higher the sucrose intake, the lower the HDL cholesterol (the "good" cholesterol) will be.

Multiple investigators have reached this conclusion (Yudkin et al., 1986; Tillotson et al., 1997; Archer et al., 1998). This means that an excess intake of refined sugar can also effect the development of atherosclerosis and coronary heart disease by its lowering effect on HDL cholesterol, which serves to transport cholesterol out of the blood vessels and to the liver for excretion. A low HDL cholesterol level means that cholesterol is tending more to accumulate in the blood vessel walls than to be taken out, consistent with the ongoing development of atherosclerosis.

Hypertriglyceridemia, another atherosclerosis risk factor discussed earlier, also appears to be directly affected by the ingestion of sucrose (Story, 1982). Smith et al. (1996) found that an average reduction of sucrose intake in the diet of greater than 70% resulted in an average reduction in plasma triglyceride levels of greater than 20%. It would appear that increased sucrose intake accounts for at least some of the elevated triglycerides found in so many people.

Increased dietary sugar also relates to heart disease and vitamin C deficiency by an indirect, yet nevertheless significant mechanism. More dental caries (cavities) are associated with a greater consumption of sucrose (Karjalainen et al., 2001). This correlation between sucrose and dental decay has also been documented in animal studies (Pekkala et al., 2000).

Until dentistry changes its current approach to dental care, more dental decay means more mercury-containing fillings (Huggins and Levy, 1999). The placement of more mercury fillings means more gum disease (Sotres et al., 1969; Turgeon et al., 1972; Trivedi and Talim, 1973) and even more periodontal disease (Fisher et al., 1984). More gum and periodontal disease means more chronic seeding of the body and the blood vessels with microbes and their metabolic toxins. As discussed under the section on inflammation, this chronic seeding also helps to assure a focal depletion of vitamin C in the arterial walls, even in the face of a reasonable intake of dietary and supplemental vitamin C. Also, severe decay can sometimes proceed directly to the performance of root canal procedures, which assures an even more potent and continuous source of vitamin C-depleting microbes and associated toxins (Meinig, 1996; Kulacz and Levy, 2002).

Therefore, refined sugar intake appears to promote the development of atherosclerosis and heart disease by a number of mechanisms. However, an induced vitamin C deficiency in the blood vessel walls through both direct and indirect mechanisms appears to be one of the very significant ways in which refined sugar exerts this pro-atherosclerosis effect.

CHAPTER 11
Smoking and Vitamin C Deficiency

Smoking is another well-established, independent, and major risk factor for the development of atherosclerosis and coronary heart disease (Frank, 1993; Menotti et al., 2004). Many, if not most, of the mechanisms by which smoking causes atherosclerosis appear to at least utilize vitamin C deficiency as a cofactor.

Bourquin and Musmanno (1953) not only found that smoking lowered the blood level of vitamin C, they also found that adding nicotine to samples of whole human blood significantly lowered the vitamin C content of that blood. Durand et al. (1962) showed that the blood levels of vitamin C in smokers were markedly reduced, and that nonsmokers generally had twice as much vitamin C in their blood as the smokers. McCormick (1957) commented that tobacco smoking is "the greatest despoiler of vitamin C." He also

> **EXHIBIT 63**
> Smoking significantly lowers vitamin C content of blood.

noted that it was found that the smoking of a single cigarette, "as ordinarily inhaled," metabolized or oxidized an equivalent amount of vitamin C in the body to that found in an average orange. Indeed, in the light of such information, it is readily apparent that a smoker of only one pack of cigarettes per day would have great difficulty in ever achieving normal body levels of vitamin C as long as only dietary and not supplemented vitamin C was ingested.

Stone (1976) cited a large number of studies in demonstrating the clear ability of tobacco smoking to oxidize vitamin C and reduce its stores in the body. Quite long ago, only shortly after the discovery of vitamin C, Strauss and Scheer (1939) showed in 25 subjects given 200 mg of vitamin C the ability of only one to three cigarettes smoked to constantly and markedly reduce the urinary excretion of vitamin C, implying its direct oxidation by the smoking and its byproducts.

The vitamin C status of even the nonsmoker is impaired by tobacco smoke in the immediate environment. Strauss (2001) examined children chronically exposed to tobacco smoke. Strauss found that even after adjusting for age, gender, vitamin C intake, and multivitamin intake, exposure to tobacco in the immediate environment remained "significantly associated" with lower blood levels of vitamin C.

Preston et al. (2003) reached a similar conclusion, finding that environmental tobacco smoke, even with "minimal" exposure, resulted in a "highly significant" reduction of plasma ascorbate levels.

McCormick further noted that in hundreds of vitamin C blood tests on smokers not a single normal level was found. Pelletier (1977) found that as a group cigarette smokers have average blood levels of vitamin C that are 30% lower than the average levels seen in nonsmokers. Furthermore, Pelletier found that those who smoke more than 20 cigarettes a day have vitamin C levels that are 40% lower than normal. In fact, Pelletier (1975) found that the decrease in the blood levels of vitamin C appeared directly proportional to the amount of tobacco smoked.

Probably the primary reason that smoking effectively consumes so much vitamin C is that it is a huge source of free radical oxidants. Maritz (1996) noted that a single puff of smoke contains 10^{15} of these oxidants.

Most likely, vitamin C exerts much of its effects due to its role as the body's primary antioxidant. When vitamin C meets free radicals, it is quenched and oxidized in direct relation to the number of free radicals that need reduction/neutralization. This is very similar to the lowering of vitamin C levels by the increased oxidant stress seen with diabetes, discussed earlier. The more an individual smokes, the more vitamin C will be immediately utilized, and the lower that individual's blood vitamin C level will go.

In citing his own earlier work (McCormick, 1945), McCormick also noted the incredible percentage of smokers among individuals who had sustained fatal heart attacks. He noted that of 151 patients who died in this manner, 97% of them had been smokers. Today, this percentage will still be high, but probably not quite as high due to the numbers of people ingesting more and more vitamin C and other antioxidants from both supplements directly and from foods that have been supplemented.

McCormick also noted that a particularly severe form of vascular disease known as Buerger's disease was always associated with smoking. Buerger's disease is associated with such rapidly progressive narrowings and blockages of the arteries that gangrene often occurs when the blood supply becomes compromised enough, resulting in amputation of fingers or toes.

Patients with this disease generally not only smoke, they smoke a lot. These patients may smoke as much as three to four packs of cigarettes (60 to 80 cigarettes) a day. In the *Cecil Textbook of Medicine* (2000) it is noted that patients with this disease who quit smoking can almost always avoid amputations, while 40% or more of patients who continue smoking will eventually have one or more amputations.

It is much more than coincidence that such an incredibly severe and rapidly progressive form of vascular disease as Buerger's disease is seen under circumstances where blood vessel content of vitamin C has to be minimal to nearly nonexistent. Not surprisingly, such patients often have coronary artery disease with the associated anginal chest pains and eventual heart attacks.

In addition to the direct effects that smoking has in lowering vitamin C levels and resulting in all of the problems that develop with such a deficiency, smoking also helps to directly promote other risk factors for atherosclerosis. And as mentioned earlier, a deficiency of vitamin C helps these other risk factors to exert their effects.

Solomon et al. (1968) found that periodontal disease is much more common in smokers than in non-smokers. Furthermore, in studying 341 individuals in a Veterans Administration hospital, Shannon (1973) found a strong correlation between lower whole blood vitamin C levels and increasing severity of periodontal disease.

As noted earlier, periodontal disease has now been found to be strongly correlated to atherosclerosis and heart attacks. Furthermore, it would appear that the ability of smoking to rapidly destroy vitamin C is probably a primary reason facilitating the development of the periodontal disease.

Cohen (1955) found that the administration of vitamin C to children with significant gum disease was able to clearly improve the condition. Gum disease virtually always precedes advanced periodontal disease, and it can be practically considered as an early form of periodontal disease. It would seem a logical conclusion that the especially severe vitamin C deficiencies seen in smokers play a significant role in causing the periodontal disease that is also independently correlated with the development of atherosclerosis and heart attacks.

Smoking is also associated with a condition of reduced blood flow that makes any established atherosclerotic narrowings more symptomatic and clinically significant. Zhang et al. (1999) found that in 23 of

24 test subjects there was a 40 to 50% decrease in the amount of blood flow in the capillaries (microcirculatory blood flow) within one to five minutes after smoking.

Reductions in this microcirculatory blood flow can result in, or help to cause, anginal chest pain and heart attack just like the blockages in the much larger arteries. However, when 2,000 mg of vitamin C was given to these subjects two hours before smoking, there was a very significant (50%) lessening of the cigarette-induced reduction of the capillary blood flow. Using the same dose of vitamin C, Teramoto et al. (2004) were also able to restore coronary microcirculatory function and the acutely impaired coronary flow velocity reserve in the smokers tested. Gamble et al. (2000) also showed that vitamin C protected against some of the cardiovascular and microvascular changes seen after cigarette smoke inhalation in man, including the overall degree of heart rate acceleration typically noted post-inhalation.

EXHIBIT 64

2 grams of vitamin C taken 2 hours prior to smoking produced 50% reduction in the restriction of capillary blood flow normally caused by smoking.

Cigarette smoking also helps to promote atherosclerosis by its activating effects on white blood cells, resulting in their clumping together and sticking to the blood vessel wall. This sticking of the white blood cells to the blood vessel wall appears to play an active role in the causation of atherosclerosis and other diseases associated with smoking (Janoff, 1985; Ross, 1993). And once the sticking has taken place, both acute and chronic damage can be inflicted on the blood vessel wall by these white blood cells (Weiss, 1989; Lehr and Arfors, 1994).

Lehr et al. (1994) found that in hamsters a vitamin C pretreatment "almost entirely prevented" this clumping of white blood cells together and their subsequent sticking to the blood vessel wall after exposure to cigarette smoke.

Furthermore, the authors noted that the plasma levels of vitamin C reached in the hamsters were easily attainable in humans by vitamin C supplementation. It should be noted, however, that in a chronic smoker the amounts of vitamin C would have to be massive to maintain an acceptably normal plasma level of vitamin C.

Nevertheless, it would appear that one more of the atherosclerosis-causing mechanisms of cigarette smoking needs a vitamin C deficiency to exert its effects.

In the discussion of cholesterol as a risk factor, the important role of LCAT was discussed. This enzyme, which helps to pull cholesterol out of the blood vessel wall by helping it to bind to HDL, is dramatically inhibited in experiments exposing human plasma to cigarette smoke (McCall et al., 1994; Bielicki et al., 1995). Furthermore, Chen and Loo (1995) showed that vitamin C helps to prevent the reduction of LCAT levels by oxidants.

Therefore, the extensive destruction of vitamin C by smoking allows a greater oxidant destruction of LCAT activity. Although an indirect mechanism, this

represents still another way in which smoking promotes atherosclerosis by the effects of the vitamin C
deficiency that it induces.

CHAPTER 12
Homocysteine and Vitamin C Deficiency

An increased level of homocysteine in the blood is yet another major and independent risk factor for atherosclerotic vascular disease (Clarke et al., 1991; Maxwell, 2000; Gupta et al., 2005; Yang et al., 2005). Omland et al. (2000) were able to show that higher homocysteine levels in acutely ill patients presenting with unstable angina or heart attack were predictive of shorter survival times.

Boers (2000) asserted that even a mildly increased level of homocysteine is a risk factor for atherosclerosis equal in strength to the risk factors of elevated cholesterol and smoking. In an analysis of 27 other studies relating homocysteine to atherosclerosis, Boushey et al. (1995) concluded that elevated blood homocysteine levels accounted for a full 10% of the population's risk for coronary artery disease.

Nygard et al. (1997) have shown that in patients with documented coronary artery disease higher blood levels of homocysteine are significant predictors of an increased chance of death. Rasouli et al. (2005) showed that elevated homocysteine levels "strongly and independently" predict the progression of atherosclerosis, as measured by increased coronary plaque burden.

Homocysteine is an amino acid that is not found in the diet, but is formed exclusively as a breakdown product of another amino acid, methionine (Hajjar, 2001).

Methionine is an essential component of the diet, and it serves as a source of sulfur for normal metabolism. Nappo et al. (1999) used a large oral dose of methionine in healthy subjects to induce a mild to moderate increase in blood homocysteine levels. They showed that this elevation in homocysteine had a significant negative impact on a number of parameters associated with early atherosclerosis, including the activation of factors associated with blood clotting and factors associated with a greater stickiness of the blood vessel lining.

Most significantly, they showed that pretreatment with vitamins C and E was able to block these effects of the induced elevated homocysteine levels. These alterations in blood clotting and blood vessel wall stickiness are likely significant factors in the way increased homocysteine levels exert their effects, as den Heijer et al. (1996) were able to show that veins will also be much more likely to get blocked with blood clots when homocysteine levels are elevated.

Another effect of an intentionally induced elevation of the blood homocysteine level is a decrease in blood flow, due to a smaller caliber of the blood vessel. Remember that arteries have muscle fibers in the vessel walls, and this musculature can relax (vasodilation) or contract (vasoconstriction), thereby affecting blood flow.

Chambers et al. (1999) were able to show that pretreatment with vitamin C was able to block the ability of an increased homocysteine level to slow blood flow by a squeezing effect of the muscle fibers in the blood vessel wall. The vitamin C was able to keep the arteries being tested in a state of vasodilation, resulting in the maintenance of greater blood flow.

Since vitamin C is such a potent antioxidant, it has been postulated that most of the above negative effects of elevated homocysteine levels are caused by increased levels of oxidant molecules, which vitamin C is capable of neutralizing.

Loscalzo (1996) noted that increased levels of homocysteine are associated with a number of different reactive molecules capable of exerting what he called "oxidative stress" on the body. Starkebaum and Harlan (1987) and Wall et al. (1980) provided evidence that some of these reactive molecules associated with too much homocysteine are capable of damaging blood vessels by such oxidative mechanisms.

Kanani et al. (1999) also noted that oxidant stress appeared to play a role in the inability of the arteries to inadequately relax (vasodilate) in the face of increased levels of homocysteine, and that oral dosing of vitamin C blocked this effect and allowed normal vasodilation.

Just as the other risk factors for atherosclerosis rarely exert their negative effects in a completely independent manner, elevated homocysteine levels can also have some effects that directly involve some of the other risk factors already mentioned.

Inflammation is a significant risk factor, and the multiple ways in which a vitamin C deficiency helps inflammation promote atherosclerosis have already been discussed. In studies with mice Hofmann et al. (2001) found that an elevated homocysteine level not only accelerates atherosclerosis, it also enhances the inflammatory process in the blood vessel.

Certainly, the effects that an elevated homocysteine level plays in making white blood cells clump together and stick to the blood vessel wall, mentioned earlier, can play a significant role in the promotion of inflammation in those affected areas.

It is also of interest to note that Hofmann et al. found that a diet rich in B vitamins (specifically: folate, B6, and B12) was able to significantly decrease homocysteine levels as well as their negative vascular effects in the mice studied. Also, in human subjects with documented coronary artery disease, Bunout et al. (2000) found that supplementation with folate and antioxidant vitamins (including vitamin C) was able to reduce blood homocysteine levels.

However, using only vitamin C supplementation (4,500 mg daily), Bostom et al. (1994) were unable to demonstrate a significant lowering effect on elevated homocysteine levels in patients with established coronary artery disease.

Diabetes, another risk factor intimately involved with chronic deficiencies of vitamin C, often also inter-relates with abnormal homocysteine metabolism.

Drzewoski et al. (2000) compared healthy control subjects with poorly controlled diabetic patients. They found that the diabetics had "significantly higher" levels of homocysteine in their blood than the controls. It is also of interest that these researchers found that the lower the circulating insulin levels were in these diabetics, the higher their homocysteine levels were.

Recall that insulin plays an important role in getting vitamin C into different cells and tissues of the body. This research can also allow an inference that lower vitamin C levels inside the cells of the body is also associated with higher circulating levels of homocysteine in the blood.

In studies of guinea pigs with scurvy, it has also emerged that vitamin C has some very specific roles in the metabolism of homocysteine. McCully (1971) concluded that oxidized vitamin C facilitates the oxidation of homocysteine in the body, which promotes the formation of a substance call homocysteic acid.

McCully was also able to conclude that homocysteic acid was important for the proper synthesis of the proteoglycan components of connective tissues, including the connective tissue components of the blood vessels.

Overall, then, it appeared that vitamin C plays an important role in allowing homocysteine to be properly metabolized and play its important role in the synthesis and maintenance of healthy connective tissues and blood vessels. When vitamin C is severely depleted, the result is not only deficient connective tissue and blood vessel walls, but also an added amount of unmetabolized homocysteine free to circulate in the blood and result in the other mechanisms of damage already discussed.

While the role that an elevated homocysteine level plays in the development of atherosclerosis is not as well defined as with some of the other risk factors, it again appears that vitamin C deficiency likely plays an integral role in maximizing the negative impact of this risk factor. However, it would also appear that a balance of other dietary nutrient factors, such as folate and vitamin B6, is also very important in the proper therapeutic approach to minimizing the impact of an elevated blood homocysteine level as a risk factor for atherosclerosis.

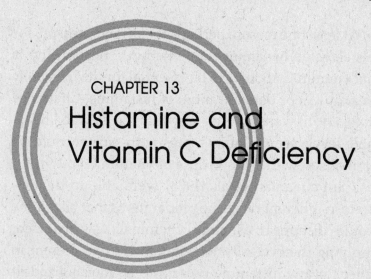

CHAPTER 13
Histamine and Vitamin C Deficiency

Although not recognized as a traditional risk factor for atherosclerosis, histamine is included here because of its likely relationship to the development of atherosclerosis, and because of its seemingly clear-cut regulation by vitamin C. Histamine is normally found in almost all of the cells of the body. When tissues are injured or when certain types of immune reactions are set in motion, histamine is often released from its storage sites. It has been shown that mast cells, which have increased concentrations of histamine, are prevalent in unstable atherosclerotic plaques (Clejan et al., 2002).

Histamine levels in the blood are inversely related to vitamin C levels in the blood (Clemetson, 1980; Johnston et al., 1992; Johnston et al., 1996). Generally, the higher the histamine level is, the lower the vitamin C level is, and vice-ver-

> **EXHIBIT 65**
>
> **Histamine levels in the blood are inversely related to blood levels of vitamin C.**

sa. At least one reason, perhaps the primary reason, for this elevated histamine/low vitamin C relationship is that vitamin C appears to be essential for the metabolic breakdown, or detoxification, of histamine. Chatterjee et al., (1975) were able to show that the elevated histamine levels seen in guinea pigs with scurvy could be normalized with a single dose of vitamin C.

Subramanian et al. (1973) were able to demonstrate in different rat tissue preparations that histamine would disappear as more vitamin C was oxidized, implying the necessity for vitamin C to be present in order for any histamine present to be metabolized. It would appear that when vitamin C levels are low, histamine then begins to accumulate due to its decreased breakdown, resulting in multiple adverse effects.

Histamine and the effects exerted by histamine are intimately involved with inflammation, another risk factor for atherosclerosis discussed earlier. Histamine excess may well be one of the more significant mechanisms involved in the promotion of atherosclerosis by inflammation.

EXHIBIT 66

Histamine has been implicated as an important regulator of cells that produce inflammatory response.

In fact, histamine has been implicated as an important regulator of some of the cells that produce the inflammatory response (Marone et al., 2001), and these cells have already been shown to play an important role in the early development of atherosclerosis (Gerrity, 1981; Brown and Goldstein, 1983).

Another effect of this released histamine is to induce a degree of separation between the walls of endothelial cells. Clemetson (1999) asserted that a chronic excess of histamine will result in a picture of "capillary fragility" such as is seen in scurvy. When clear zones of separation are seen surrounding the endothelial cells in a network of capillaries, at least some degree of increased "capillary fragility" can be anticipated as well.

Gore et al. (1965) were able to demonstrate under the electron microscope that endothelial cells lining the aortas of guinea pigs with scurvy had definite zones of separation between them ("diastasis"), versus the normal state of adjacent cell walls appearing to be in direct contact.

Earlier, Majno and Palade (1961) had already demonstrated that histamine administration would cause similar zones of separation between cells in rats, as visualized under the electron microscope. When such zones of separation appear between endothelial cells, the dissolved substances in the blood, including cholesterol, have increased access to the internal lining of the blood vessel, and abnormal depositions can begin.

Majno et al. (1961) asserted that plasma actually escapes through these gaps between the cells. The basement membrane is then forced to serve as a filter, directly promoting the deposition of cholesterol and other atherosclerotic blood solutes in that area of the vessel wall. Also, recall that vitamin C deficiency directly alters the nature of the basement membrane itself, further predisposing to these initial cholesterol/lipid depositions.

Chronically elevated levels of histamine are at least one reason, and perhaps a primary reason, that the endothelial lining of the artery becomes more permeable, or porous, allowing an easier deposition of cholesterol into the arterial wall to initiate the development of atherosclerosis.

In a rabbit tissue model, DeForrest and Hollis (1980) were able to show that histamine appeared to play a definite role in the initiation of atherosclerosis by increasing blood vessel wall permeability. Also working with rabbits, Owens and Hollis (1979) were able to demonstrate that a variety of stresses associated with increased atherosclerosis were able to stimulate the formation of histamine directly on-site in the blood vessel wall, further implying that histamine is a significant factor in the initiation of the atherosclerotic process.

EXHIBIT 67

Antihistamine drugs shown to inhibit the development of atherosclerosis.

Even more support for the atherosclerotic properties of histamine comes from studies with chlorpheniramine, an antihistamine. Antihistamine drugs counteract the actions of histamine in the body. Harman (1961) was able to demonstrate that chlorpheniramine could inhibit the development of atherosclerosis in rabbits fed a high cholesterol diet.

Hollander et al. (1974) were able to achieve similar results in rabbits fed a high cholesterol diet and given chlorpheniramine. They were able to specifically show that the antihistamine-treated rabbits had less lipid deposition in the arterial walls, along with a lesser degree of cellular proliferation than is usually seen in developing atherosclerosis. At the very least, excess histamine appears to have a contributory role in the development of atherosclerosis. However, Clemetson (1999) makes a case for excess histamine being "the most likely cause" for the development of atherosclerosis.

Since a severe enough vitamin C deficiency keeps the histamine levels elevated in the blood, it would appear that a chronic vitamin C deficiency can account for still another biochemical mechanism that can contribute to both the initiation and the ongoing development of atherosclerosis.

CHAPTER 14

Infection and Vitamin C Deficiency

Infection, like elevated histamine levels, is not a generally recognized risk factor for atherosclerosis. However, infection can seed microorganisms throughout the body, with some ending up in the blood vessel walls. When this occurs on a chronic basis, a secondary chronic inflammation can be expected to ensue, and atherosclerosis can be expected to develop by the mechanisms already discussed above under the risk factor of inflammation.

An infection does not have to be chronic to result in the provocation of heart disease. Meier et al. (1998) conducted a large, population-based study to examine the association between the risk of heart attack (myocardial infarction) and the occurrence of recent acute respiratory tract infection, such as the common cold. They found that people did have an increased risk of heart attack (three-fold higher) when they had an acute upper respiratory tract infection in the previous

10 days. Furthermore, the authors made this finding in a population "without a history of clinical risk factors" for heart attack.

Although the authors did not look at blood or tissue vitamin C levels, the one thing that such an infection (typically viral) does is to dramatically and acutely decrease vitamin C levels in the body. Hume and Weyers (1973) found that cold viruses were highly effective in acutely lowering vitamin C levels in humans. They found that after only the first two days of a cold, a 50% decrease in the levels of vitamin C in the white blood cells was observed.

EXHIBIT 68

Viral RNA found in arteries of victims who died of myocardial infarction.

More recently, enteroviral RNA was detected in approximately 17% of the 128 human atherosclerotic vascular lesions examined (Kwon et al., 2004). Also, Kotronias and Kapranos (2005) found herpes simplex viral DNA in the coronary arteries of 38% of 42 individuals dying of myocardial infarction.

Frei et al. (1990) asserted that vitamin C is the most effective antioxidant in human blood plasma.

EXHIBIT 69

Infections rapidly neutralize body stores of vitamin C.

These researchers also noted that infections stimulate the formation of a number of oxidants, or reactive oxygen species, which can kill the invading microorganisms. However, too many oxidant molecules for too long a period of time, as in chronic infections, will eventually do damage to the various cells of the body as well. In the absence of adequate vitamin C supplementation, a vicious cycle of infection-induced vitamin C deficiency combined with an infection-induced increased production of oxidant molecules can initiate or aggravate a number of diseases, of which atherosclerosis is only one. This relentless cycle can only really be broken when enough supplemental vitamin C is taken to neutralize the oxidant molecules, eradicate the infection, and stop the ongoing production of more oxidant molecules and the ongoing depletion of vitamin C stores that resulted directly from the infection.

In light of the extensive data already presented on the impact of vitamin C deficiency on the development of atherosclerosis, one logical conclusion from the information just presented is that an acute vitamin C deficiency can destabilize preexisting atherosclerotic narrowings.

Discussed at greater length in the section on myocardial infarction, a syndrome known as unstable angina frequently precedes the actual heart attack. Vita et al. (1998) found a strong correlation between low blood levels of vitamin C and the appearance of unstable angina. This is strong support for the supposition that a substantial vitamin C deficiency can significantly increase the risk for sustaining a heart attack.

Certainly, the presence of an infection that rapidly metabolizes vitamin C can utilize at least this one mechanism in allowing an atherosclerotic plaque to destabilize and block off completely, leading to heart attack.

CHAPTER 15
Coronary Artery Calcium and Vitamin C Deficiency

The presence of calcium deposits in the coronary arteries is now known to be an independent predictor of premature coronary heart disease (Taylor et al., 2005). These researchers showed that among young, asymptomatic men the mere presence of coronary artery calcium was associated with an 11.8-fold increased risk for coronary heart disease. Also, among those individuals who had coronary artery calcification, they were also able to show an increasing risk of coronary heart disease with increasing degrees of calcification. In a recent epidemiological study Simon et al. (2004) demonstrated a higher prevalence of coronary artery calcium in men with "low to marginally low plasma ascorbic acid levels."

EXHIBIT 70

Presence of calcium deposits in coronary arteries associated with over 1000% increase in risk for Coronary Heart Disease.

The study of Simon et al. noted above correlating more coronary artery calcium with lower levels of vitamin C is not really surprising when the literature addressing the relationship between vitamin C and calcium metabolism is examined. Calcium is the most abundant mineral in the body, and it is found in nearly all of the organized tissues in the body. Combined with phosphate, it forms calcium phosphate, the hard, dense material found in bones and teeth. Calcium is also important in its dissolved, ionic form, as it is essential for the normal beating of the heart and for the normal functioning of muscles and nerves. Furthermore, calcium is an integral part of the blood clotting mechanism, and many enzymes need calcium to function properly.

Bourne (1942), in looking at the role that vitamin C plays in the repair of injured tissues, noted that scurvy, the ultimate deficiency state of vitamin C, seemed to be associated with an increased excretion of calcium and a tendency not to be deposited in bone.

EXHIBIT 71

Atherosclerosis-like calcium deposits found to be abnormally deposited in various tissues of individuals with scurvy.

Rather, Bourne noted that calcium had been found to be abnormally deposited in various tissues in scurvy in an unorganized, "amorphous" form, similar to the calcium deposits seen in atherosclerosis. This would suggest that severe vitamin C deficiency allows calcium to be mobilized from its large reservoir in the bone and to be excreted in greater amounts, as well as to be redeposited elsewhere.

Such a mechanism would appear to favor the development of osteoporosis (thinned-out, brittle bones) and lessened bone mineral density. In fact, Morton et al. (2001) found that postmenopausal women who took vitamin C supplements had greater bone mineral density. Hall and Greendale (1998) also found higher bone mineral density in postmenopausal women with greater dietary vitamin C intake.

EXHIBIT 72

Postmenopausal women who supplement with vitamin C found to have greater bone mineral density.

Melhus et al. (1999) looked at 66,651 female smokers and concluded that inadequate dietary intake of vitamins C and E probably increased the risk of hip fracture in these women. Leveille et al. (1997) found that women from 55 to 64 years of age who had supplemented vitamin C for 10 years or longer and had not taken estrogens had a higher bone mineral density than non-supplementers of vitamin C in the same age range.

As a more general correlation, Falch et al. (1998) found that elderly patients who fractured their hips had a "significantly lower" level of vitamin C in the blood than elderly patients who had not sustained such a fracture.

In guinea pig studies, Poal-Manresa et al. (1970) found that even though vitamin C deficiency did not absolutely prevent the formation of new bone, enough of a deficiency did prevent good quality new bone from being formed.

Salter and Aub (1931), in earlier guinea pig studies, found that a diet adequate in calcium but deficient in vitamin C prevented deposition of the calcium into the bone. They also were able to show the subsequent addition of vitamin C back into the diet allowed calcium to be "rapidly deposited."

The mobilization of calcium from the bones secondary to vitamin C deficiency also strongly suggests an additional mechanism in which atherosclerosis is promoted. After vitamin C deficiency causes calcium to come out of the bone, some of it will then be free to abnormally deposit in susceptible areas of the blood vessels before being excreted, thereby directly promoting the development of atherosclerosis.

EXHIBIT 73

Vitamin C is incredibly effective in dissolving calcium and keeping it in solution.

Another reason that vitamin C deficiency plays such a significant role in abnormal calcium metabolism relates to the incredible ability of vitamin C to dissolve calcium to a very high concentration. Ruskin (1938) found that calcium carbonate, normally one of the most difficult substances to dissolve regardless of the dissolving agent, could be rapidly and completely put into solution with vitamin C. Ruskin noted that the completeness of the dissolving ability of vitamin C was "second only to fairly strong hydrochloric acid."

Ruskin also commented on the uniqueness of a relatively weak biologic acid such as vitamin C to be able to singularly dissolve calcium carbonate so effectively.

Overall, the scientific literature shows that vitamin C is intimately involved in calcium metabolism in the body. Consistent with the epidemiological study of Simon et al. (2004) noted above, a vitamin C deficiency appears to strongly promote the dissolving out of calcium from the bone while facilitating its abnormal redeposition into the arteries, directly facilitating coronary artery calcification, another established coronary heart disease risk factor.

CHAPTER 16

Copper, Iron, and Vitamin C Deficiency

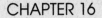

COPPER

A high copper status in the body, as reflected by an elevated level of copper in the blood, is another independent risk factor for the development of atherosclerosis and coronary heart disease. Salonen et al. (1991) conducted a study on 2,655 men over about a 57-month period. The men with the highest serum copper levels (upper third) had nearly a six-fold greater incidence of heart attacks than the men with the lowest serum copper levels in the study group.

> **EXHIBIT 74**
>
> **Men with highest serum copper levels found to have 600% greater incidence of heart attack than men with the lowest serum copper levels.**

Similarly, Harman (1963) was able to demonstrate significantly higher serum copper levels in volunteers with a history of heart attack versus volunteers who did not have a history of heart attack. He suggested that lowering serum copper levels "by dietary or chemical means" was a reasonable course of action to decrease the probability of development of atherosclerotic heart disease.

Other researchers have also found that increased levels of copper in the body are significantly related to heart disease. Manthey et al. (1981), looking at patients examined by X-ray dye studies (angiography), found higher serum copper levels in patients with severe blood vessel disease versus those with no disease.

Kok et al. (1988), looking at both heart disease and cancer, found a four-fold increased risk of death from these conditions in those members (upper one-fifth) of a study group of 10,532 who had the highest serum copper levels, relative to those with normal levels.

EXHIBIT 75

Individuals with highest serum copper levels found to have 400% greater risk of death from cancer or heart disease than individuals with normal levels.

Punsar et al. (1975) were able to demonstrate an increased 10-year mortality from heart attack to be associated with an increased content of copper in the drinking water.

Finally, Singh et al. (1985) were able to demonstrate some interesting findings relating serum copper to heart attack severity. They found that mean peak serum copper levels were "significantly higher" in clinically complicated cases of heart attack versus uncomplicated cases. Furthermore, they found that serum copper levels showed a "highly significant" rise over the first seven days after a heart attack, with a gradual decline to normal by the 28th day after the heart attack.

It would appear that an elevated copper level not only predisposes to a heart attack, it may also predispose to, or directly contribute to, some of the complications seen with a heart attack.

Salonen et al. (1991) theorized that one of the mechanisms by which increased copper promoted heart disease was its ability to inactivate selenium. Selenium is a trace metal inversely related to risk of heart attack, as demonstrated in a prospective study (Salonen et al., 1982). Lower selenium levels were associated with higher rates of heart attack in this study.

Another mechanism by which copper could promote atherosclerosis is by its ability to promote the oxidation of LDL cholesterol (Heinecke et al., 1984; Palinski et al., 1990). Steinberg et al. (1989) asserted that oxidized LDL cholesterol likely increases the ability of LDL cholesterol to promote atherosclerosis.

Carr et al. (2000) also asserted that oxidized LDL is a definite factor in the formation and activation of atherosclerotic lesions.

> **EXHIBIT 76**
>
> **Ceruloplasmin, the protein that carries copper in the blood, oxidizes vitamin C, thereby reducing the level of beneficial vitamin C in the blood.**

Perhaps the most significant mechanism by which increased copper levels promote atherosclerosis is through the metabolic destruction/oxidation of vitamin C. The protein that carries copper in the blood, ceruloplasmin, acts to oxidize, or metabolize, vitamin C (Humoller et al., 1995; Osaki et al., 1964), thereby reducing the levels of unoxidized (reduced), beneficial vitamin C in the blood.

Furthermore, when there is less reduced vitamin C available in the blood and tissues, the copper that is present can more readily help to oxidize LDL cholesterol, mentioned above. In other words, when there is less reduced vitamin C available to donate its electrons (oxidize) to copper, the copper will seek its electrons elsewhere, resulting in a greater oxidation of LDL cholesterol.

Jialal et al. (1990) examined this likely interplay between vitamin C and copper in the oxidation of LDL cholesterol. They found that vitamin C appeared to inhibit this copper-mediated oxidation. Therefore, the more that copper can directly lower the unoxidized vitamin C levels in the body, the less unoxidized vitamin C is available to inhibit the oxidation of LDL cholesterol by copper.

Animal studies have also supported the concept that copper can use up the active form of vitamin C. Szoke et al. (1963) found that the administration of a simple copper salt (cupric sulfate) reduced the vitamin C content in the liver and adrenal glands of guinea pigs. Mazur et al. (1960) were also able to show that providing copper in the cupric ion form (Cu++) was able to facilitate the oxidation of vitamin C in preparations of rat liver.

Overall, then, an excess of copper and/or copper-containing proteins appears to be a risk factor for the development of atherosclerosis. A deficiency of the physiologically active, reduced form of vitamin C (ascorbic acid) appears to be at least one of the significant mechanisms by which excess copper exerts this effect.

IRON

Iron is another substance associated with an increased risk of heart attack when present in excess (Shah and Alam, 2003). Salonen et al. (1992) were able to demonstrate that excess ferritin, a primary form in which iron is stored in the body, was associated with an increased risk of heart attack in the Finnish men they studied. This finding received further support in epidemiological studies looking at serum ferritin levels, increased risk of coronary artery disease, and myocardial infarction (You and Wang, 2005).

> **EXHIBIT 77**
>
> **Serum ferritin (iron) levels greater than 200 mcg/liter associated with a 220% greater risk of heart attack.**

Specifically, a serum ferritin level at or greater than 200 micrograms/liter was associated with a 2.2-fold greater chance of heart attack than in the men with a lower serum ferritin. These researchers also used a model that adjusted out for many of the other common factors that would also be associated with an increased risk of heart attack.

Also, like copper, a water supply overloaded with iron is also associated with increased oxidative stress (Rehema et al., 1998). Increased oxidative stress is associated with the oxidation of lipids, which makes them more likely to contribute to the development of athersclerosis. Furthermore, a primary role for vitamin C is to combat and neutralize increased levels of oxidative stress.

When iron stores are high and vitamin C stores are already low, the general balance in the body leans more toward oxidation than reduction, and the levels of active vitamin C are pushed even lower. And, regardless of the reason vitamin C levels are low, atherosclerosis will develop more readily under such conditions.

Minqin et al. (2003) studied newly formed atherosclerotic lesions in rabbits fed a high cholesterol diet. Some of the rabbits were also given desferrioxamine, an iron-chelating agent. The rabbits that were on the desferrioxamine for the longest time showed reductions in the progression of their atherosclerotic lesions. Furthermore, when the more extensive lesions in both the control and desferrioxamine-treated animals were analyzed, a higher concentration of iron and a lower concentration of zinc were found. The authors hypothesized that the early atherosclerotic lesions in their animals might be accelerated by free radical production secondary to increased iron levels, and that the zinc might help neutralize that effect.

Overall, then, this study is reasonably good evidence that iron is a promoter of atherosclerosis. The information known on the ability of iron to be a promoter of oxidation also suggests that adequate levels of antioxidants, such as vitamin C, would be a significant factor in preventing the induction of atherosclerosis by iron. Conversely, it also suggests that a vitamin C deficiency would be a strong promoter/accelerator of the pro-atherosclerotic effect of iron.

Another very good study that looked at iron content and vitamin C levels was conducted by Lynch et al. (1967). These investigators found that the adult Bantu population of South Africa had a high incidence of iron overload in their bodies. Furthermore, they found that this same population had an exceptionally high incidence of scurvy.

EXHIBIT 78

Population with high incidence of scurvy also found to have high incidence of iron overload in their bodies.

In an earlier study it had already been noted that the majority of patients in this population with scurvy did have excess iron stores (Bothwell et al., 1964). It therefore seemed logical to Lynch et al. that the iron overload seen in many Bantus might well be the direct cause for the severe deficiencies of vitamin C being seen. They found that the administration of vitamin C to Bantus with excess iron stores, relative to normal control subjects, resulted in a more rapid disappearance of the vitamin C from the blood, along with the increased presence of the primary breakdown product of vitamin C in the urine. This directly indicates that excess iron likely accelerates the metabolic breakdown of vitamin C.

Shah and Alam (2003) summarized nicely the mechanistic evidence for the role of iron in atherosclerosis. They noted that:

- Iron has a role in the oxidation of low-density lipoprotein (LDL),

- Iron chelators prevent the endothelial cell damage induced by oxidized LDL,
- Iron itself has the ability to directly induce endothelial cell damage,
- Iron chelators prevent endothelial cell dysfunction and the proliferation of vascular smooth muscle, and
- Iron appears to have a role in the causation of myocardial reperfusion injury.

It would appear that iron is a metal that readily promotes the oxidation and subsequent metabolic breakdown of many different molecules, including vitamin C. As such, it is a very significant factor in the development and/or maintenance of a vitamin C deficiency in the body, both by directly inducing the oxidation of vitamin C and by using up vitamin C stores that help prevent and/or restore the oxidative damage rendered to other molecules (Valko et al., 2005). Such a vitamin C deficiency can then independently promote the development of atherosclerosis and coronary heart disease through the other mechanisms previously noted.

CHAPTER 17
Oxidative Stress and Vitamin C Deficiency

There has also been increasing evidence that a metabolic state generally favoring oxidation (versus reduction) is a likely contributor to the development of atherosclerosis. This has been characterized as a state of increased "oxidative stress." Gackowski et al. (2001), looking at one of the typical biomarkers of oxidative stress, found that patients with higher levels of this biomarker in the blood lymphocytes had lower levels of vitamin C. This is not surprising, since vitamin C remains the most powerful reducing agent (antioxidant) known to occur naturally in living tissues (Cameron, 1976; Frei et al., 1990).

> **EXHIBIT 79**
> Vitamin C is the most powerful antioxidant known to occur naturally in living tissues.

Increased oxidative stress as a risk factor for atherosclerosis clearly overlaps with, and is intimately involved with, a number of different risk factors already discussed (Frei, 1999). These risk factors include hypertension, cholesterol, homocysteine, inflammation, diabetes, smoking, infection, copper, and iron, which all involve an increased free radical presence in the development of atherosclerosis. An increased presence of free radicals in the body and the blood vessels is another way to describe a state of increased oxidative stress. Regardless of what is causing the increased oxidative stress, a relative deficiency of vitamin C must always exist to allow this risk factor to exert its effects. Although other antioxidants can combat oxidative stress, they would likely never be completely effective in neutralizing this factor in the presence of a severe enough vitamin C deficiency.

EXHIBIT 80

The appearance of oxidative stress always requires a relative deficiency of vitamin C for this risk factor to exert its harmful effects.

CHAPTER 18
Physical Activity and Vitamin C Deficiency

Decreased physical activity is also recognized as a risk factor for the development of coronary heart disease (Clemetson, 1999). The ability of exercise to reduce the risk of such disease remains poorly explained. However, Fishbaine and Butterfield (1984) did a very interesting study looking at the vitamin C status of joggers versus a sedentary group. Although the study size was small, they found that blood vitamin C levels were significantly higher in men who ran 10 miles a day versus the same men who later ran only five miles a day. Furthermore, relative to individuals who were non-exercisers consuming the same dietary amounts of vitamin C, the runners still maintained significantly higher vitamin C blood levels. The reasons for these findings are not clear. However, the authors do

> **EXHIBIT 81**
> Exercisers maintain significantly higher vitamin C levels than non-exercisers who consume identical amounts of dietary vitamin C.

note that the runners excreted less vitamin C in their urine, possibly indicating that the kidneys tended to conserve and retain more vitamin C. The authors still did not think this explanation was adequate to explain the degree of difference in vitamin C levels in the compared groups.

Regardless of the explanation, it would appear that there is some support in the literature to assert that exercise exerts at least some of its beneficial effects on the reduction of heart disease and atherosclerosis by maintaining increased levels of vitamin C in the body.

CHAPTER 19
Obesity and Vitamin C Deficiency

Obesity is another risk factor for atherosclerosis and heart disease (Correia and Haynes, 2004). Obesity, defined here as an increase of 20% above ideal body weight, is generally related to an increasing incidence of other atherosclerosis risk factors, including high blood pressure, elevated blood cholesterol, diabetes, and physical inactivity. Reinehr and Andler (2004) showed that weight loss in obese children favorably modified the "atherogenic profile," which they defined as hypertension, reduced HDL cholesterol, increased LDL cholesterol, increased tryglycerides, and insulin resistance.

This is strong supportive evidence that the obesity itself helps provoke and/or maintain the presence of some of the most clear-cut cardiovascular risk factors. Cassidy et al. (2005) have shown that obesity is positively associated with coronary artery calcification, which has already been noted above to be an independent indicator/risk factor of the presence and extent of coronary atherosclerosis. Also, Ogawa et al. (2004) have demonstrated that obesity is a risk factor for the development of the type of vascular disease seen in diabetes.

EXHIBIT 82

Vitamin C
deficiency is a
significant factor
in the expression
of all risk factors
associated with
obesity.

Similarly, Singhal (2005) has noted that childhood obesity appears to be "associated with endothelial dysfunction and greater arterial stiffness from as early as the first decade of life." Singhal also noted that "weight loss is beneficial" for this condition. As already discussed earlier, vitamin C deficiency is a significant factor in the expression of all these risk factors.

CHAPTER 20
Season and Vitamin C Deficiency

Although it may seem a bit odd at first, the likelihood of having a hospitalization for coronary heart disease seems to vary according to the time of the year. Multiple investigators have found that heart attacks occur significantly more often in the winter months than in the summer months (Sher, 2000; Spencer et al., 1998; Ornato et al., 1996; Douglas et al., 1995; Enquselassie et al., 1993). Arntz et al. (2000) were able to demonstrate a greater incidence of sudden death during the winter months, a finding that would certainly correlate significantly with a greater incidence of heart attack.

EXHIBIT 83

Heart attacks occur significantly more often in the winter months than in the summer months.

Other investigators have looked at the seasonal variation in vitamin C levels in the body. Lenton et al. (2000) looked at the levels of vitamin C in white blood cells (lymphocytes), finding as much as 38% higher levels when cells were examined in the summer months versus the winter months. Dobson et al. (1984) also found the highest vitamin C levels in the blood and white blood cells in the summer months, with the lowest levels seen in the winter months. It would appear, then, that the seasonal variation of heart attack incidence relates inversely to vitamin C levels. When vitamin C levels are down in the winter months, heart attacks are more frequent, and when the vitamin C levels rise in the summer, heart attacks lessen in number.

EXHIBIT 84

Vitamin C levels in the blood and in white blood cells are significantly lower in the winter than in the summer.

The reasoning behind the variation in vitamin C levels in the body relative to the time of the year has to do with the availability of fresh fruits and vegetables. Fresh produce is less available in the winter and much more available in the summer. When people do not supplement vitamin C and they have a limited budget to buy produce that has been shipped into their area of the country, vitamin C levels can be expected to drop significantly during the winter months.

EXHIBIT 85

Vitamin C supplementation found to counteract seasonal decline in vitamin C levels.

Furthermore, produce that needs to be shipped will contain lower amounts of vitamin C than produce that is consumed locally directly after its harvest. Significantly, although probably not surprisingly, Zheng et al. (1989) were able to demonstrate that vitamin C supplementation was able to counteract the seasonal decline in vitamin C levels.

Similarly, Dobson et al. (1984) were able to show that a small dose of vitamin C abolished the rise in serum cholesterol levels seen in the winter. As discussed earlier, elevated cholesterol levels in the blood will typically result from a vitamin C deficiency and serve as a risk factor for the development of heart disease and atherosclerosis.

Further support for this seasonal modulation of heart attack frequency relating to vitamin C levels comes from the work of Ku et al. (1998). They found that in a subtropical area without temperature extremes no seasonal variation in the incidence of heart attacks could be found.

Subtropical areas have vitamin C-rich produce available year-round, and it does not suffer any of the vitamin C depletion seen with storage and shipping. It is unlikely that the people living in such an area will have the variations of vitamin C in their bodies that are seen in the people living in areas where all such produce must be shipped in during the winter months, generally with a price tag that further limits the volume of consumption for the general public.

Not surprisingly, heart attack incidence for the aged during the winter months is higher than for younger individuals (Sheth et al., 1999). As noted earlier, the elderly will also tend to have lower vitamin C levels independent of the time of the year. Therefore, the two factors together, age and season, should be expected to at least be additive in their associations with lower vitamin C levels and higher rates of heart attack.

CHAPTER 21

Depression, Psychosocial Factors, and Vitamin C Deficiency

Depression is a mental state in which there exists a mood characterized by feelings of sadness, despair, and discouragement. As discussed here, depression will refer to what is known as endogenous depression. Endogenous depression implies that a biological cause rather than an environmental cause exists. In contrast, a reactive depression would be the direct result of a stressful life event, just as might be seen after the death of a spouse or other beloved family member.

Depression has emerged as an independent risk factor for coronary heart disease (Malhotra et al., 2000; Rowan et al., 2005). It is also a predictor of poor prognosis for patients who have already had heart attacks (Rowan et al., 2005) Ferketich et al. (2000), while controlling for possible confounding factors, found that depression was associated with an

> **EXHIBIT 86**
> Depression linked to higher incidence of coronary heart disease in men and women.

increased incidence of coronary heart disease in both men and women.

Other investigators have reached similar conclusions, although their studies took slightly different angles. Cohen et al. (2001), after controlling for other known cardiovascular risk factors, found that a history of treatment for depression was "significantly associated" with the subsequent occurrence of heart attack. Ariyo et al. (2000), looking specifically at elderly Americans, found that symptoms associated with depression appeared to be an independent risk factor for the development of coronary heart disease and mortality from all causes.

Vaccarino et al. (2001) looked at the effects of depression on the outcome of heart failure patients. Heart failure can be associated with coronary disease and atherosclerosis, but not necessarily so. They found that an increasing number of depression-related symptoms relates to a worsened prognosis for patients with heart failure. Greater numbers of such symptoms predicted a higher risk of functional decline or death from the heart failure. Parissis et al. (2005) found that depression is as much as four to five times as common in heart failure patients.

A number of investigators have found that psychosocial factors such as a type A personality, increased anxiety and stress, or increased hostility are associated with a greater incidence of coronary heart disease. A type A personality is one that is characterized as highly competitive and ambitious, seeming to constantly struggle with the surrounding environment. Such a personality could also be considered as being largely equivalent to a situation of chronic stress.

Appels et al. (1987) and Appels et al. (1982) found that individuals with type A behavior "tended to have higher incidences of angina pectoris." Cohen et al. (1979) also demonstrated a slightly greater

EXHIBIT 87

A-type personality associated with higher incidence coronary heart disease.

incidence of coronary heart disease among Japanese Americans with a type A personality relative to those without one. Jenkins (1982) also noted that anxiety and depression, as well as a type A personality, appear to correlate "with a variety of manifestations of coronary heart disease." Zyzanski et al. (1976) found that men who demonstrated evidence of greater depression and anxiety on testing also had more advanced atherosclerosis on their angiograms. The angiograms were read independently of the behavioral testing.

Kubzansky and Kawachi (2000) looked at the effects of depression in concert with anger and anxiety. In a review of articles published between 1980 and 1998 they were able to conclude that "growing evidence indicates that negative emotions may influence the development" of coronary heart disease. More specifically, they found that the evidence implicating anxiety in the onset of such heart disease was the strongest, while the association between anger and heart disease was "limited but suggestive."

They also noted that depression was consistently linked to an increased chance of death following heart attack. Kubzansky et al. (1998) also looked at anxiety more specifically as a risk factor for heart disease. They reviewed papers published between 1980 and 1996 on anxiety and coronary heart disease, concluding that anxiety "may contribute to the risk" of developing coronary heart disease.

Kubzansky et al. (1997) also looked at worry as a more specific component of anxiety and concluded that high levels of worry may also increase the risk of coronary heart disease in older men.

Siegman et al. (2000) studied dominance as a personality trait and how it correlated with coronary heart disease risk. Their data suggested that dominance, regardless of anger level, was an independent risk factor for coronary heart disease in older men. Siegman et al. (2000a) also looked at hostility as another psychosocial factor and found that their data indicated hostility was yet another "significant" independent risk factor for coronary heart disease. Breaking down their test results further, they found that irritability was the specific trait in their profiling that correlated significantly with coronary heart disease.

EXHIBIT 88

Anxiety, stress, hostility, worry, irritability, dominance, and anger all tied to development of atherosclerosis and risk of heart attack.

Viewing the above information collectively, it would appear that depression and a host of psychosocial factors are clearly related to the development of atherosclerosis and the risk of heart attack.

These psychosocial factors include a type A personality, anxiety, stress, hostility, worry, irritability, dominance, and anger. We will now see that all of these factors, along with depression, appear to become most pronounced when toxin levels and cholesterol levels are highest and vitamin C levels are lowest.

We will also see that this occurs because depression and all of the other factors already mentioned are typically the clinical manifestation of unneutralized toxins. And when these toxins remain unneutralized, cholesterol levels tend to be highest and vitamin C levels tend to be lowest. Enough supplemental vitamin C can also be expected to largely eliminate the presence of these risk factors and their negative effects on the development of heart disease.

As discussed earlier in the section addressing cholesterol as a risk factor for heart disease, both vitamin C and cholesterol serve to help inactivate a variety of different toxins. High cholesterol levels generally reflect a high level of circulating toxins that need inactivation. This implication has been drawn in both human and animal studies (Bloomer et al., 1977; Alouf, 1981; Chi et al., 1981; Tarugi et al., 1982; Huggins and Levy, 1999; Alouf, 2000).

Huggins (1993) pointed out that most of his patients who had mercury fillings in their mouths and were being chronically exposed to this toxic heavy metal also had a typical array of symptoms. Among other symptoms,

> **EXHIBIT 89**
> **Depression and irritability related to toxins — especially mercury leached from amalgam dental fillings.**

most of the patients also had significant depression and irritability. Removal of the mercury often resolved these symptoms. Also, a prospective study looking at baseline and follow-up blood testing demonstrated that the removal of the mercury fillings was noted to consistently result in the lowering of previously elevated baseline cholesterol levels (Huggins and Levy, 1999).

As also noted earlier in the section on cholesterol, low cholesterol levels also have been shown in multiple studies to be strongly correlated with an increased chance of getting cancer or dying from cancer (Kark et al., 1980; Williams et al., 1981; Kagan et al., 1981; Stemmermann et al., 1981; Keys et al., 1985; Gerhardsson et al., 1986; Schatzkin et al., 1987; Knekt et al., 1988; Isles et al., 1989; Cowan et al., 1990).

One very good explanation for this is that when circumstances exist so that existing toxins are not adequately neutralized, the immune system faces much greater chronic challenges, and cancer can eventually result. This reasoning of unneutralized toxicity due to low levels of cholesterol could also explain some otherwise seemingly inconsistent findings.

Kalinina et al. (1993) found there was also an increased risk of death from heart attack in men with low blood levels of both total cholesterol and LDL cholesterol.

Rodriguez (2001) also reported that both high and low cholesterol levels were associated with increased coronary heart disease risk. She found that a cholesterol of 240 mg% or higher was associated with a 90% increased risk of developing heart disease, while a cholesterol level below 160 mg% was associated with a 55% increased risk of developing heart disease. It would appear that high cholesterol levels certainly directly accelerate the process of atherosclerosis, but low cholesterol levels mean not enough protection exists to protect against a variety of toxins, which will also directly lead to accelerated atherosclerosis.

Generally, a high cholesterol level means the toxic problem is still there, but the body is making a valiant compensatory effort to deal with the issue. When cholesterol-lowering medications are taken or too much dietary deprivation of cholesterol-containing foods is experienced, cholesterol levels can drop even though the toxic presence is still there.

As just mentioned above, significant diseases such as cancer can then result. Moreover, existing depression can progress to suicide (Golomb, 1998; Golomb et al., 2000). In a similar fashion, other preexisting psychosocial behaviors such as hostility, irritability, or anger can progress to acts of violence when cholesterol levels become lowered.

In one subset of college males, Greene et al. (1995) were able to demonstrate that the traits of aggressiveness and dominance were associated with increased levels of total serum cholesterol. Many such patients will also be found to have significantly depleted levels of vitamin C in blood and tissues, and aggressive vitamin C supplementation can help to substantially eliminate these psychosocial behaviors.

Several authors have provided evidence that a symptom like depression is associated with something causing the heart disease and is not just "naturally" resulting from the psychological consequences of having a serious, life-threatening disease. Jonas and Mussolino (2000) were able to show that depressive symptoms are also associated with an increased risk of having a subsequent stroke. This alone is strongly suggestive that the depression is a marker indicating the presence of unneutralized toxicity in such patients, as such toxicity could then account for the increased chance of having a stroke.

Carney et al. (1999) were also able to show that the effective drug therapy of depression in patients who had a heart attack did not reliably decrease subsequent cardiac symptoms or chance of cardiac death. This result again strongly implies that the depression is resulting from something else (like toxins) and eliminating the depressive symptoms with drugs does not eliminate the toxicity that caused the depression in the first place.

Under such circumstances the toxins will remain unneutralized and free to accelerate the progression of heart disease, as well as other diseases. It has also been suggested by some researchers that depression could be associated with platelet activation (Roose and Spatz, 1999; O'Connor et al., 2000), which could then be associated with more heart attacks as the platelets help to provoke the clotting associated with the acute expansion of preexisting arterial plaques. Once again, unneutralized toxicity could easily be the cause of platelets becoming more prone to sticking together and causing new clots.

Depression has also been shown to respond therapeutically to the administration of vitamin C (Cocchi et al., 1980). These researchers demonstrated in a five year-old girl that the depression associated with the administration of steroids could be relieved by vitamin C. This is not especially surprising since steroid administration will reliably metabolize and help to use up vitamin C stores. However, they also reported on three additional patients, a seven year-old child, a 19 year-old, and a 29 year-old. All three were considered to have a depression of unknown cause.

> **EXHIBIT 90**
> Vitamin C supplementation shown to produce complete recovery in some cases of depression.

They were given daily intravenous vitamin C at a dosage of 50 mg/kg/day. The authors reported that all three patients had "complete recovery from mental disturbances." This gives further strong support to the hypothesis that an agent, such as a toxin, can be causing the depression. When enough vitamin C is administered, the toxin is neutralized and the depression lifts. When the depression is treated in this manner rather than with any of a variety of antidepressant drugs, the initial depression should also cease to be a risk factor for heart disease, since the culprit toxins are also being neutralized by the vitamin C.

> **EXHIBIT 91**
> Depression appears to accelerate metabolism of vitamin C.

It should also be noted that depression appears to be one more condition that accelerates the metabolism of vitamin C. In an animal research model felt to cause depression in rats, Blake-Mortimer et al. (1998) showed that the tissue vitamin C levels fell significantly, by 20% to 30%. Such a concept is important since it would indicate that the administration of vitamin C is needed to keep depression from further lowering vitamin C levels, even if the initial depression had nothing to do with a vitamin C deficiency.

The bulk of the evidence examining depression and other psychosocial risk factors for atherosclerosis and heart disease indicates that unneutralized toxicity (as is often seen with multiple mercury amalgam fillings) is probably the primary reason that these risk factors are present in the first place. As already discussed in the section on inflammation as a risk factor for heart disease, toxins are enormously effective in metabolizing and using up vitamin C stores.

Whenever there is enough toxicity present to cause these risk factors to emerge, it can also be anticipated that a substantial, if not very severe, vitamin C deficiency will also be present as well. As such, vitamin C deficiency is likely an important, or even primary, reason that depression and the other noted psychosocial factors have been documented to be risk factors for atherosclerotic heart disease.

CHAPTER 22
Heart Rate and Vitamin C Deficiency

Recent research has established that the heart rate is an independent predictor of not only cardiovascular, but also noncardiovascular and overall mortality in middle-aged males (Seccareccia et al., 2001).

These investigators studied 2,533 Italian men aged 40 to 69 years. They found that a higher heart rate not only predicted a higher rate of heart death, it also was one of the most important independent predictors of overall mortality, all other risk factors being equal. They found that the risk of death increased about 50% for each 20-

EXHIBIT 92

Elevated heart rates a very important predictor of heart death, and overall mortality as well.

beat-per-minute increment increase of heart rate. They also found that the relative risks between the extremes of heart rate evaluated were more than 2-fold. In overall agreement with these findings, Palatini and Julius

(2004) have asserted that an elevated heart rate is a "major" risk factor for cardiovascular disease.

While there can be any of a number of different reasons why one's heart rate would be faster than normal, a deficiency of vitamin C is one of them. In studying guinea pigs, Sankaran and Krishnan (1936) established that a vitamin C-deficient diet, designed to cause scurvy, would ultimately resulted in a marked increase in heart rate. They noted that the average guinea pig heart rate was between 250 and 275 beats per minute. The animals deprived of vitamin C would accelerate their heart rates to a range of 300 to 375 beats per minute. They also noted that a rapid heart rate ("tachycardia") was clinically observed to occur in human scurvy.

EXHIBIT 93

Tachycardia (rapid heart rate) clinically observed in human scurvy.

While there can exist other reasons for a rapid heart rate in a given patient, it appears likely that a significant depletion of vitamin C is at least one significant contributor to the occurrence of this finding. It would be very interesting to see what levels of vitamin C were present in the blood and white blood cells of the patients studied by Seccareccia et al. who eventually died, compared to those who survived. This could help to clarify how important the vitamin C level is in affecting significant increases in the heart rate.

CHAPTER 23
Fibrinogen and Vitamin C Deficiency

Fibrinogen is the main protein involved in the clotting mechanism in the blood plasma, and it also factors directly into how viscous ("thick") the blood is. Fibrinogen can also play a role in how readily the platelets in the blood will stick together and promote the initiation of blood clots. Fibrin, a very important component in the blood clot, results from the direct conversion of fibrinogen when the clotting mechanism in the blood has been initiated.

An increased level of fibrinogen in the blood is an independent risk factor for cardiovascular disease (Kannel et al., 1987; Tunstall-Pedoe et al., 1997; Nyyssonen et al., 1997; Bielak et al., 2000; Paramo et al., 2004).

EXHIBIT 94

Abnormally high levels of fibrinogen in the blood increases risk for cardiovascular disease.

An elevated fibrinogen level in the blood can be expected to increase both the likelihood of a gradual increase in the size of atherosclerotic plaques as well as the likelihood of sudden complete blockages by acutely formed blood clots on top of developing plaques.

Khaw and Woodhouse (1995) were able to demonstrate a strong and consistent relationship between fibrinogen and vitamin C levels in the blood. Higher fibrinogen levels were seen with lower levels of vitamin C. Hume et al. (1982) looked at patients who had sustained a stroke, finding that, following such

EXHIBIT 95

Low levels of vitamin C in the blood related to higher levels of fibrinogen.

an event, blood fibrinogen levels were up and blood vitamin C levels were down. Generally, patients who have a stroke have sudden blockages of brain blood vessels at diseased sites in the arterial walls, just as heart attack victims have sudden blockages in their coronary arteries supplying the heart muscle.

While a vitamin C deficiency appears to be directly associated with an increased chance of the blood clotting due to increased fibrinogen levels, vitamin C also appears to play a critical role in the dissolving of blood clots already formed. This ability to dissolve blood clots is known as fibrinolytic activity. Bordia et al. (1978) looked at the acute effects of vitamin C administration

EXHIBIT 96

Vitamin C supplementation increases ability to dissolve clots.

on the fibrinolytic activity levels in both healthy individuals as well as individuals with coronary artery disease. They found that the administration of only 1,000 mg of vitamin C by mouth produced a significant elevation of the ability to dissolve blood clots in both of these groups. They also noted that this effect of vitamin C persisted only as long as the increase of vitamin C in the blood persisted, indicating the importance of maintaining the increased level. Interestingly, the same daily dose of vitamin C was found to help prevent excessive fibrinolysis in patients with chronic nephritis, demonstrating that vitamin C, overall, appears to be important in maintaining the balance between fibrin formation and fibrin breakdown, when one effect or the other is too dominant (Shimizu et al., 1970).

Another study supportive of a vitamin C deficiency as being causative of an increase in fibrinogen levels comes from the work of Iso et al. (1996). They concluded that women exposed to passive smoking probably increased their risk of heart disease due to increased fibrinogen levels. Although such a study is very indirect in supporting this relation between vitamin C deficiency and increased fibrinogen levels, smoking has already been noted to be one of the greatest consumers of vitamin C. Any smoke exposure, whether active or passive, can be expected to have a significant effect in lowering vitamin C levels, which would then be expected to result in raised fibrinogen levels.

Fibrinogen appears to be a risk factor that involves a vitamin C deficiency in exerting its effects as a heart disease risk factor. At the very least, there is a clear correlation between elevated fibrinogen levels and decreased vitamin C levels. It is also very possible that the vitamin C deficiency itself directly results in the elevation of the fibrinogen levels in the body.

CHAPTER 24

White Blood Cells and Vitamin C Deficiency

High white blood cell (WBC) counts are emerging as another coronary risk factor (Ensrud and Grimm, 1992; Manttari et al., 1992; Gillum et al., 1993; Capuano et al., 1995; Nyyssonen et al., 1997; James et al., 1999; Brown et al., 2001; Piedrola et al., 2001). However, a significant amount of literature is continuing to emerge indicating that high WBC counts are just another indicator of increased inflammation, which has already been discussed as its own coronary risk factor.

EXHIBIT 97

Elevated white blood cell levels are associated with increased inflammation, which is another important coronary risk factor.

Elevated WBC levels have been associated with periodontitis, an inflammation/infection known to be associated with increased risk of coronary disease (Inoue et al., 2005).

Increased WBC levels have also been associated with the low-grade chronic inflammation and early cardiovascular risk in women with polycystic ovary syndrome (Orio et al., 2005).

Also supporting the role of an increased WBC count as a risk factor for coronary artery disease or just an additional indicator of ongoing inflammation are the studies that have correlated this increased count with increased mortality in patients with preexisting coronary artery disease (Haim et al., 2004), increased cardiac events in patients with peripheral coronary artery disease (Haumer et al., 2005), and just increased amounts of ischemia in patients who are postinfarction but asymptomatic (2003).

These are all conditions already strongly associated with increased levels of inflammation in the arterial system. Green et al. (1996) even found that an increased WBC count is an independent laboratory predictor of acute myocardial infarction, the ultimate clinical manifestation of progressive atherosclerosis.

Also, as already noted, a state of vitamin C deficiency favors the development and maintenance of infection and inflammation, both conditions that are strongly associated with the presence of elevated white blood cell counts. Therefore, it is to be expected that the presence of adequate vitamin C in the body is at least one significant factor that will help prevent white blood cell counts from becoming elevated.

CHAPTER 25

Coronary Artery Spasm and Vitamin C Deficiency

Coronary artery spasm is a condition in which the arterial blood vessels supplying blood to the heart muscle go into various degrees of vasoconstriction, or spasm. When the muscle in the arterial wall contracts the actual caliber of the blood vessel is decreased, and the downstream blood flow is decreased as well. It is also important to realize that this spasm can range from minimal, with little effect on blood flow, to dramatic, with a complete blockage of blood flow.

Even when the spasm completely blocks off the blood flow, the spasm will typically ease off in a few minutes. However, such spasm sometimes will not ease off readily, and the patient can have a significantly-sized heart attack, even with coronary arteries that show no obvious narrowings on angiogram (X-ray dye injected into the blood vessel).

It is also important to know that even though coronary artery spasm can affect the larger caliber coronary arteries, as noted above, it can also affect the small blood vessels not visualized on angiogram (microvascular spasm). This form of spasm will not usually cause a heart attack, but it will decrease the blood flow in enough of the heart muscle that typical heart-related anginal chest pain can result.

As noted earlier in the risk factor section on Lp(a), Pauling (1991, 1993, and 1993a) reported on two patients with significant atherosclerotic blockages in their coronary arteries responding very well to vitamin C and lysine. However, a third patient had no visible blockages on angiography, and the clinical response (reduced anginal chest pain) was just as dramatic. The positive responses resulted within two to four weeks on initiating therapy, which probably would not have been enough time to allow a substantial physical de-bulking of any obstructing atherosclerotic plaques chronically present in the arteries.

Also as noted earlier, Kaufmann et al. (2000) were able to show that vitamin C reverses the decreased blood flow typically seen in the small blood vessels of smokers.

There is a strong presumption here that it was the relief of microvascular spasm of small blood vessels that was being reversed. Supporting this presumption, Kugiyama et al. (1998) were able to directly provoke severe spasm of the larger coronary arteries with a spasm-inducing agent (acetylcholine), documented by angiography. When they infused vitamin C selectively into a specific coronary artery and then added an infusion of acetylcholine while the vitamin C infusion continued, no spasm could be induced. Furthermore, these researchers discovered that increased levels of free radicals were present in the coronary arteries of the patients with induced coronary artery spasm. An increase in the free radical load represents a source of increased oxidant stress, as discussed earlier, and suggests that coronary artery spasm may be provoked by such stress, preventable by the antioxidant properties of vitamin C.

Vitamin C has also been documented to be effective in increasing the blood flow in the veins, which have far less muscle content than the arteries. Grossman et al. (2000) showed that vitamin C could dilate (open up) the veins in the hands of human subjects, but they were uncertain about the mechanisms involved.

EXHIBIT 98

Vitamin C shown to be effective in increasing blood flow in veins by dilating those vessels.

However, regardless of the mechanisms involved in the relaxation of vascular musculature by vitamin C, all heart patients should be on sizeable daily doses of vitamin C. Keeping the muscle tone as relaxed as possible in the blood vessels, diseased or not, will help any patient to have as optimal a blood flow in those arteries as possible. This will help to minimize the clinical consequences of any atherosclerotic narrowings that are already present.

CHAPTER 26

Myocardial Infarction and Vitamin C Deficiency

Myocardial infarction, the medical term for a heart attack, occurs when the blood supply to an area of heart muscle is blocked or compromised for a long enough period of time that some death of heart muscle tissue takes place. The most common reason for a heart attack taking place is when a coronary artery supplying blood to a portion of the heart either becomes critically narrowed, or the existing atherosclerotic plaque becomes disrupted, activating local blood clotting mechanisms and blocking off the artery completely (Rauch et al., 2001). Additionally, varying degrees of coronary artery spasm, discussed in the previous chapter, can make any coronary artery narrowing suddenly critical at any time, also resulting in a heart attack if the spasm persists long enough.

The clinical syndrome that often ends up in a heart attack is known as unstable angina. Patients may present with a picture of anginal chest pain attacks increasing in frequency and duration for hours to weeks prior to the heart attack. Vita et al. (1998) found that low blood levels of vitamin C independently predicted the presence of this unstable angina syndrome.

EXHIBIT 99

Low blood levels of vitamin C independently predict the presence of the unstable angina syndrome which often precedes heart attacks.

They felt that their data indicated that antioxidant therapy played a role in lessening the degree of "lesion activity" in critically situated atherosclerotic plaques. In other words, they felt that vitamin C made arterial narrowings more stable, with a decreased likelihood of rupture and the resulting formation of an obstructive blood clot in the artery.

Research has been done looking at the effects of vitamin C and other antioxidants on the size of heart attacks. In one double-blind, placebo-controlled trial Singh et al. (1996) looked at the effects of a combined regimen of beta-carotene and vitamins A, C, and E. The vitamin C dose was only 1,000 mg daily. In any patient who presented with a suspected acute heart attack, the above combined regimen or a placebo was then administered for a 28-day period.

EXHIBIT 100

Post-heart attack patients taking antioxidant formula with 1,000 mg of vitamin C had better heart function, less angina and fewer heart rhythm abnormalities.

The researchers found that patients in the treated group had better heart function, along with less angina and heart rhythm abnormalities. They concluded that a combination of antioxidants could afford protection against larger heart attacks and greater complication rates.

In patients who are placed on cardiopulmonary bypass while undergoing heart surgery limited degrees of heart damage can be expected, since a machine has never been able to completely substitute for the natural function of the heart while it is paralyzed. Because of this phenomenon some investigative teams have looked at the protective effects of vitamin C on limiting the extent of this heart injury.

Westhuyzen et al. (1997) gave 750 IU of vitamin E for seven to ten days before surgery and only 1,000 mg of vitamin C one time 12 hours before surgery. They found that there was no measurable reduction in heart damage resulting from the operation.

However, Dingchao et al. (1994) looked at the effects of vitamin C at a dose of 250 mg/kg before undergoing heart surgery with cardiopulmonary bypass.

EXHIBIT 101

A mega dose of vitamin C prior to bypass surgery produced significant protection of the heart.

This dose, which translates to 17,500 mg of vitamin C for a 150-pound person and 23,300 mg of vitamin C for a 200-pound person, did show significant protection of the heart.

Relative to the group that did not receive vitamin C, the treated group had significantly lower cardiac enzyme levels. Lower cardiac enzyme levels mean less heart damage. Furthermore, the hearts in the vitamin C-treated group demonstrated better recovery (spontaneous recovery of beating without electrical shock) after surgery than the hearts in the untreated group. Just as is seen with the effective vitamin C treatment of infectious diseases (Levy, 2002), the dose of vitamin C must also be significant in amount to see a protective effect against heart muscle damage. 1,000 mg of vitamin C in a single dose, as given above by Westhuyzen et al., is an inconsequential amount to protect against the incredible stress of stopping the heart and operating on it.

Mickle et al. (1989) deliberately blocked one of the primary coronary arteries (left anterior descending) in dogs for two hours, and then allowed blood flow to return for another four hours. They were able to show that infusions of vitamins C and E were able to significantly reduce the sizes of the heart attacks provoked by the blocking of this coronary artery.

Similarly, Laskowski et al. (1995) randomly administered an infusion of mannitol with 10,000 mg of vitamin C in people presenting with heart attacks. In 42 patients the vitamin C infusion was given with clot-dissolving therapy, and in another 42 patients only the clot-dissolving therapy was given. These investigators found that the added vitamin C therapy was effective in reducing some of the complications associated with heart attacks.

In another animal study antioxidant therapy that included vitamin C was able to lessen the degree of damage sustained in heart attacks. Klein et al. (1989) treated pigs with vitamins C and E before blocking off their left anterior descending coronary arteries. The blockages were reversed after 45 minutes, followed by

72 hours of restored blood flow. A significant reduction in the amount of heart damage was seen in the pigs given the vitamin combination.

At least one reason why vitamin C is effective in reducing the size of a heart attack and the incidence of associated complications relates to the potent antioxidant effects of vitamin C.

Dusinovic et al. (1998) measured the activity of a number of different important antioxidative enzymes in patients who sustained heart attacks. They also measured these enzyme levels at varying periods of time after clot-dissolving therapy was administered to these patients, which opens up the blocked coronary artery and restores the blood flow to the heart in most cases.

They compared their results to the results found in 30 healthy volunteers. They found that a greater level of oxidative stress was present both immediately after heart attack and also after the clot-dissolving therapy administered for heart attack.

Ozmen et al. (1999) also found an increase in the free radical content of the blood in heart attack patients after clot-dissolving therapy. Simpson and Lucchesi (1987) wrote a review article supporting the concept that an increased free radical load in the blood after coronary artery blockage and subsequent re-opening plays a significant role in causing more pronounced cellular injury and a larger heart attack.

It would appear that the potent properties of vitamin C as an antioxidant can help to counteract this increased oxidative stress, lessening both heart attack size and complication rate by at least this one mechanism.

Another likely reason why vitamin C is effective in reducing both the size of a heart attack as well the chance of complications comes from its ability to affect protein synthesis (Gudbjarnason et al., 1966).

In dogs that had some of their coronary arteries intentionally tied off, vitamin C was found to dramatically stimulate the synthesis of new protein in the middle of the areas of heart muscle most affected by the loss of blood supply. Two separate infusions of 2,000 mg of vitamin C in the first 24 hours after the deliberately induced heart attacks were administered. In four dogs so treated, an average of a 122% increase in protein synthesis was seen in the middle of the heart attack site.

Even more significantly, the authors noted that this increase in protein synthesis was achieved in spite of the fact that the study animals had no signs of an overall vitamin C deficiency. Precise vitamin C levels were not reported, however.

This information is especially significant since vitamin C is already known to be essential for the proper formation of adequate amounts of significantly strong scar tissue, which contains sizeable amounts of collagen (Pirani and Levenson, 1953).

It would appear that vitamin C, particularly when considering damaged muscle tissue, is especially useful in the healing process, since it helps in the synthesis of both protein (muscle) tissue as well as strong scar tissue.

Gudbjarnason and his co-researchers also noted that a significant stimulation of cardiac muscle protein synthesis after experimental heart attack seemed to be associated with a lower incidence of subsequent aneurysm formation. An aneurysm is a very weakened area that outpouches from the heart wall, just like a weakened area in a bicycle inner tube. Such an area can no longer contract and presents a risk for early rupture, an almost uniformly fatal event.

Heart attacks are most likely to occur in people with narrowings already present in the arteries of the heart (coronary heart disease). Ramirez and Flowers (1980) found that the levels of vitamin C in the white blood cells were significantly lower in such people than in those without documented atherosclerosis of the heart arteries.

Generally, lower vitamin C levels in the white blood cells are felt to more accurately represent tissue stores of vitamin C than just lower levels of vitamin C in the blood. Hume et al. (1972) even asserted that a low enough vitamin C level in the white blood cells can be equated to a state of "subclinical scurvy." Such a finding should come as no surprise, however, in light of all the information presented so far indicating the significance of a vitamin C deficiency in the evolution of coronary atherosclerosis leading to heart attack.

EXHIBIT 102

Scurvy-like levels of vitamin C found in post-heart attack patients 12 hours after attack.

The lowered vitamin C levels in the white blood cells continue to decline even further after a heart attack. Hume et al. (1972) found that the depletion of vitamin C in the white blood cells bottomed out to scurvy-like levels within 12 hours after heart attack in the patients tested. They also found that the decline in vitamin C did not relate to the severity of the heart attack. Machtey et al. (1975) found after heart attack that there were "highly significant lower levels" of vitamin C in the blood on post-heart attack days two to five, compared to post-heart attack days six to eight.

These declines in vitamin C levels after heart attack strongly imply a greater need for vitamin C due to its accelerated metabolism during this period. Chamiec et al. (1996), also hypothesizing the significant contribution made by unneutralized oxidative free radical molecules to the typical full development of a heart attack, looked at the effects of vitamins C and E on the electrocardiogram (ECG).

They found that the typical deterioration in the ECG associated with an increased incidence of ventricular arrhythmias after a heart attack can be blocked by vitamins C and E. Such arrhythmias can result in sudden death in the heart victim. Chamiec et al. also found that their experimental data indicated that an increased oxidative stress was playing a significant, if not primary, role in the development of a more abnormal ECG.

EXHIBIT 103

Typical deterioration in ECG after a heart attack can be blocked by vitamins C and E.

Many ECG abnormalities that develop as the patient gets older never disappear and are largely regarded as permanent changes. Generally, such changes either remain the same once they appear, or they gradually evolve into more pronounced changes. Shafar (1967) reported on the ECG findings in two patients with scurvy before and after treatment with vitamin C.

Shafar noted that both patients had ECG abnormalities "of a degree which could be interpreted as evidence of significant myocardial disorder," even though neither patient was known to have heart disease. After seven days of vitamin C therapy, the ECGs of these two patients had essentially returned to normal.

One of the patients had very pronounced ST segment depression and T wave abnormalities. This raises the question as the whether these ECG reversals to normalcy are due to a neutralization of surrounding oxidant stress by vitamin C.

Although this question cannot be conclusively answered either way in this particular study, this would appear to be one more indication that adequate vitamin C dosing is critical in helping to maintain the health and clinical stability of the cardiac patient.

Seymour and Sowton (1964) were also able to show that vitamin C did have effects on the ECG. Two of ten medical student volunteers were given digitalis until the characteristic effects of this agent (ST flattening with T wave inversion) appeared on the ECG. 1,000 mg of vitamin C was given intravenously and improvement was seen after only 15 minutes, with a full restoration to the original normal appearance by two hours. However, these authors were not able to show any effects of vitamin C on the ECGs of patients with heart disease given digitalis. Of course, this does not rule out vitamin C having a significant effect on such ECGs if given at higher doses for longer periods of time. Furthermore, the evidence of Chamiec et al. cited above would suggest that any improvements in the ECG induced by vitamin C are truly indicative of a more healthy and stable heart.

A procedure commonly performed today to prevent a narrowed heart artery from progressing to a complete blockage and a heart attack is known as coronary artery angioplasty. This procedure involves the careful placement of a tiny uninflated balloon across a narrowed area in the artery. Upon inflation, the narrowed area is typically opened up enough so that blood flow to the heart increases, and the danger of imminent heart attack is lessened.

However, this procedure has long been plagued by a significant occurrence of re-narrowing of the blood vessel over the subsequent months. Furthermore, the re-narrowing sometimes proceeds to a greater degree of narrowing than the blood vessel had in the first place. When this happens, the patient then needs to have another balloon procedure or a heart bypass surgery, as indicated clinically.

Vitamin C also appears to be of help in the management of the balloon angioplasty patient. Tomoda et al. (1996) found that only 500 mg of vitamin C per day in 50 patients who had undergone this procedure resulted in an incidence of re-narrowing that was "significantly less" than that seen in 51 control patients. Leite et al. (2004) have demonstrated that the sites of angioplasty in blood vessel wall show persistent low-grade oxidative stress. Furthermore, they also showed that the administration of vitamins C and E led to less narrowing in the process of healing with overall improved vessel caliber.

EXHIBIT 104

Vitamin C supplementation after angioplasty shown to reduce re-narrowing of arteries.

Other investigators have also shown that antioxidants other than vitamins C and E have been successful in lessening restenosis and improving long-term clinical outcomes after balloon angioplasty (Tardif et al., 2002; Tardif et al., 2003; Lemos et al., 2005), further supporting the concept that ongoing oxidant stress (Diaz-Araya et al., 2002; Piatti and Monti, 2005) plays an important role in preventing a successful outcome after this procedure.

It would be of great interest to know what benefit even larger doses of vitamin C and other antioxidants would offer these patients.

Buffon et al. (1999) were able to show that the re-narrowing of the coronary artery after angioplasty appeared to be related to how pronounced the inflammatory response was after the procedure.

As discussed earlier in Chapter 4, inflammation is a powerful factor in the development of atherosclerosis in the first place, and it is of no surprise that it plays an important role in the re-narrowing of lesions after successful angioplasty.

Also as noted earlier, vitamin C plays a variety of roles in lessening inflammation and its impact on the atherosclerotic process. Furthermore, the nature of the inflammatory process also helps to induce more local oxidant stress. These are all good reasons why vitamin C has been noted to lessen the re-narrowing of angioplastied arteries.

CHAPTER 27
Heart Failure and Strength of Heart Contraction

As with any other muscle in the body, the muscle tissue in the heart can eventually deteriorate or become compromised and result in the clinical syndrome of congestive heart failure (CHF). In this syndrome, the heart is unable to pump blood at a level sufficient to meet the basic needs of the body's tissues. The causes of this syndrome are many. Largely due to this variety of possible causes, any given patient with CHF may have anywhere from little or no reponse to vitamin C therapy to a dramatically positive response.

An inflammation of the heart muscle tissue is one reason for developing CHF. Bearing this in mind, it is of interest to look at the

EXHIBIT 105

Scurvy, by itself, can cause myocarditis, an inflammation of the heart muscle.

work of Taylor (1937). He studied guinea pigs with scurvy and found out the scurvy alone could cause myocarditis, or inflammation of the heart muscle. He also found that guinea pigs with scurvy and infected with certain bacteria would eventually develop "congestion of the lungs and liver," a condition representing some of the clinical findings of CHF. Additionally, he noted that curing the scurvy would prevent the development of CHF. At least in the guinea pig, it would appear that severe vitamin C deficiency is one reason for developing CHF.

Also, while not a commonly reported finding, a case report was published in which a patient with scurvy presented with an enlarged heart and generalized edema (Singh and Chan, 1974). The response to vitamin C therapy "was dramatic and remarkable," and by the fourteenth day of therapy the heart size was normal on chest x-ray and the syndrome of heart failure had completely resolved.

EXHIBIT 106

Patient with scurvy, an enlarged heart and edema has complete remission after 14 days of vitamin C therapy.

Vitamin C may also benefit patients with CHF because of its diuretic action. A diuretic action means the ability to increase urine output, typically resulting in an excretion of excess fluids that have accumulated in and around the tissues of the body. Such fluid accumulation is nearly always part of the CHF sydrome.

Abbasy (1937) showed that daily vitamin C doses of 700 mg or less increased the volume of urine in the children he tested. He also noted that the diuretic effect did not appear until the body stores of vitamin C were "in a normal degree of saturation." It should also be noted that this diuretic effect of vitamin C did not require the presence of gross swelling anywhere in the body. Presumably, this diuretic effect can occur in individuals with a normal balance of fluids in their bodies. Shaffer (1944) looked at the effects of vitamin C on patients who did have swelling (edema) in their extremities. He was also able to demonstrate a "small diuresis" in the ten patients he treated. While not a profound clinical effect, this diuretic property of oral vitamin C is nevertheless a positive property of vitamin C in the treatment of the CHF patient.

In an experiment in which patients were monitored closely with catheters (tubes) inserted into their hearts, Mak and Newton (2001) were able to determine that vitamin C could play a role in making the heart contract, or squeeze, more effectively. In the presence of dobutamine, an agent known to significantly improve the ability of the heart to contract, vitamin C was able to further augment this contracting ability.

Interestingly, the vitamin C had no comparable effect on contractility in the absence of the dobutamine. Both the vitamin C and the dobutamine were directly infused into the coronary (heart) arteries. While no clear conclusion can be taken from this data as to the effect of vitamin C on a weak, failing heart, it would appear that vitamin C would likely be a positive factor in this situation as well.

CHAPTER 28
Vitamin C and Heart Health: The Statistics

Although a great deal of evidence has already been presented demonstrating the undeniable link between vitamin C deficiency and atherosclerotic heart disease, an enormous amount of statistical scientific literature also exists supporting this connection. Collectively, the results will corroborate what has already been discussed at some length: The lower your vitamin C blood and tissue levels go, the greater your chances of developing significant heart disease.

One of the best and most compelling studies was published by Khaw et al. (2001). They found that vitamin C depletion was not only associated with increased heart disease, it was also associated with an increased mortality from all causes. This is hardly surprising, as vitamin C's effects on the intercellular ground substance, as well as on the immune system, affect all cells, not just those lining the arteries supplying blood to the heart. More specifically, Khaw et al.

found that the subjects with the top one-fifth vitamin C
levels had only half the risk of death compared with

EXHIBIT 107

**Subjects with the
greatest levels of
vitamin C shown
to have half the
mortality risk of
subjects with lowest
levels.**

the subjects with the bottom one-
fifth vitamin C levels. Furthermore,
the relationship with mortality between these top and bottom levels
of vitamin C was continuous. This
means any improvement in vitamin C status could be expected to
lessen overall mortality to at least
some definable degree.

Also, significantly, these researchers found this
effect of vitamin C levels on total mortality to be independent of age, systolic blood pressure, blood cholesterol, cigarette smoking, and diabetes. Finally, as a
very practical point, these researchers concluded that
the increase in plasma vitamin C seen by increasing
the daily dietary intake of fruits and vegetables by
only about 50 grams could result in a 20% reduction in
all-cause mortality risk.

Many other studies have demonstrated a statistical benefit for the protection against heart disease by
vitamin C, although each study took its own relatively
unique angle in how data was gathered and analyzed.
Loria et al. (2000) found that men with serum vitamin C levels less than 28.4 micromole/liter had a 57%
higher risk of death from any cause, not just cardiac,
than men with greater than approximately a three-fold
higher serum vitamin C level, 73.8 micromole/liter.

Enstrom et al. (1992) found an overall reduction
in death from all causes, including cardiovascular dis-

ease, to be associated with an increased dietary intake of vitamin C. Other studies demonstrating that increased dietary intake of vitamin C reduces the chances of heart attack include the work of Fehily et al. (1993), Gey et al. (1993), Sahyoun et al. (1996), and Joshipura et al. (2001). Lynch et al. (1996) reviewed a number of studies and concluded that in animal studies "there is good evidence" of the ability of vitamin C to "slow the progression of experimental atherosclerosis."

Some studies have looked at the combined effects of vitamin C with other antioxidants on the risk of death from heart disease. Knekt et al. (1994), after correcting for the major nondietary risk factors for heart disease, found that increased dietary intake of antioxidant vitamins protects against coronary heart disease.

Riemersma et al. (1991) found that low plasma concentrations of vitamins E and C and carotene were associated with an increased risk of angina pectoris, the clinical syndrome that can often end in death from heart attack.

Carr et al. (2000), looking at the combined effects of vitamins C and E, concluded that an optimum vitamin C status in the body would likely help protect against atherosclerosis, while vitamin E was likely to be primarily effective against atherosclerosis only in combination with vitamin C.

Losonczy et al. (1996), also looking at the combined effects of supplemented vitamins C and E, found a lower risk of both total mortality and death from heart attack. Rajasekhar et al. (2004) looked at serum antioxidant levels other than vitamin C and found that higher vitamin E levels correlated with less coronary artery disease in the South Indian population that they studied. This is additional evidence that while vitamin C is very important in the prevention of heart disease, a balance of antioxidants in the body is important as well.

Cheraskin et al. (1974) looked at the effects of vitamin C on the symptoms of heart disease rather than on the more clear-cut result ultimately associated with progressive heart disease, mortality or death. They were able to conclude that cardiovascular symptoms and findings declined as daily vitamin C intake was increased. They felt that the evidence suggested that vitamin C was "a resistance agent for cardiovascular disease" since the administration of vitamin C "tends to discourage the appearance of cardiovascular symptomatology."

EXHIBIT 108

Cardiovascular symptoms and findings declined as daily vitamin C intake increased.

While the statistical study cited above (Khaw et al., 2001) is a large (30,466 subjects) prospective study that produced very compelling results on the value of vitamin C in decreasing the risk of death from coronary heart disease, the definitive study on the value of vitamin C and heart disease is yet to be done.

As with so many of the other areas of clinical vitamin C research, the dosing of vitamin C, whether through diet, supplementation, or both, remains minimal.

The most compelling data should result when, depending upon bowel tolerance (bowel tolerance is determined by steadily increasing vitamin C intake until one experiences diarrhea), roughly 6,000 to 12,000 mg of vitamin C is given daily in three or more divided doses.

All participants except those with enormously high daily toxin loads should almost completely arrest, and even often reverse, the development of atherosclerosis. However, the evidence presented in this section should be more than enough to convince even the most skeptical individuals that finding their bowel tolerance doses of vitamin C and taking them on a daily basis for life just might be good medicine.

Section Three

Responding to the Overwhelming Evidence

CHAPTER 29
Practical Suggestions for Stopping/Reversing Atherosclerosis

Is there really a way to stop your heart artery narrowings from continuing to progress? Even better, is there a way to open up your existing heart artery narrowings without surgery or angioplasty? Practically speaking, is this disease of atherosclerosis actually preventable and even reversible?

I believe the answer to all three of the questions above is a resounding "yes," and I will now present a protocol that has the potential to make atherosclerosis in most individuals a completely curable disease, or condition.

It is very important to emphasize that it is strongly recommended that all aspects of the protocol be followed closely. Some people may experience a clear clinical success after following just the supplemental aspects of the protocol, but I must emphasize that I believe the scientific evidence indicates that most people will have to follow the entire protocol, especially with regard to the proper removal of the sources of dental toxicity.

PROTOCOL FOR THE PREVENTION AND REVERSAL OF ATHEROSCLEROSIS

A. TOTAL DENTAL REVISION

Removal of dental toxicity, or Total Dental Revision, requires the following:

- Proper removal of root canal-treated teeth
- Proper treatment of chronic periodontal disease
- Proper cleaning of all cavitations
- Proper extraction of acutely and chronically abscessed teeth
- Proper replacement of mercury amalgam fillings and other toxic fillings with optimally biocompatible materials
- Proper replacement of toxic dental metals used in crowns and other dental reconstructions with optimally biocompatible materials
- Proper removal of dental implants

As discussed earlier, the presence of root canal-treated teeth ("root canals") and advanced periodontal disease in the mouth are two very strong consumers of antioxidant stores by virtue of the chronic infections and chronic toxicities associated with these dental entities.

Huggins and Levy (1999) and Kulacz and Levy (2002) have addressed the scientific and clinical evidence showing why root canals and periodontal disease are so reliably associated with a very high incidence of atherosclerosis, cancer, and other chronic degenerative diseases.

Issels (1999) noted over 50 years ago that cancer was strongly correlated with the presence of root canal-treated teeth. Cancer is a prototypical chronic degenerative disease, and the same chronic lack of antioxidant defenses found in such patients is also seen with chronic heart disease (atherosclerosis) and other chronic metabolic and degenerative diseases such as diabetes, collagen vascular diseases, osteoarthritis, and osteoporosis.

The only way to begin the proper restoration of health in a heart patient is to properly extract all root canal-treated teeth. This involves more than mere extraction. The bony sockets must be properly cleaned after the extraction of the teeth, or chronically infected holes (cavitations) will reliably form and remain after superficial healing has closed over the holes.

These toxic pockets of infection in the jawbone are pathologically identical to wet gangrene, and they have essentially the same toxicity as the root canal-treated teeth themselves. This is also why so many edentulous patients have clinical pictures consistent with large ongoing toxic challenges. When their jawbones are properly explored, even many years after the extractions took place, long channels of toxic cavitation are routinely found, as adjacent pockets often expand to the point that they merge, forming literal tunnels of gangrene in the mouths of many older patients.

This topic, as well as the proper dental techniques needed to revise cavitations and extract root canal-treated teeth, is addressed in greater detail by Kulacz and Levy (2002). The technical issues involved in cavitation surgery are also addressed by Levy and Huggins (1996).

Chronic periodontal disease has much associated infection and toxicity. This again results from the metabolism of aerobic bacteria and other microbes trapped in an anaerobic, or at least significantly oxygen-deprived, environment. Addressing chronic periodontal disease first requires that the smoking patient stop this habit.

Subsequently, the regular use of a high-intensity water irrigation device over all the gum surfaces and interfaces with bone will rapidly resolve many cases of periodontal diseases, even when advanced. It is best to use about a cup of warm water along with several teaspoons of 3% hydrogen peroxide in the container that feeds the irrigation device. A splash of mouthwash can also be added if desired for a better taste.

When first using the water irrigation on the diseased gums, ready bleeding can be expected even at the lower pressure settings. This bleeding is to be expected and should not deter continued use of the device. The irrigation should be performed two to three times a day. Most patients will notice little or no bleeding after only a few days to a week of this therapy, and frequently the highest pressure settings can then be used indefinitely.

The growth of new gum tissue can usually be noted within the first week or two of this therapy as well. This irrigation therapy as described above is also advisable for most people for the maintenance of gums that are already clinically healthy. Also, most individuals who use this therapy regularly will not require regular dental flossing, which can repeatedly traumatize the gums when not done absolutely correctly and which rarely cleans more effectively than the dental irrigation device used regularly and properly.

Another source of great dental toxicity is the acute or chronically abscessed tooth. Such a tooth poses the same toxic challenges to the body and its antioxidant status as the root canal-treated tooth, the cavitation, or the chronically infected gums. Such a tooth needs prompt extraction, followed by the proper cleaning out of the socket, in the same way as following the extraction of a root canal-treated tooth. Other measures should also be taken to minimize the acute toxicity of extracting such a tooth, discussed in further detail by Kulacz and Levy (2002).

It is also best that an individual minimize overall dental toxicity by undergoing a cleaning at all sites of suspected cavitation. Practically speaking, this boils down to cleaning at the sites of previous extractions, done in the traditional fashion not involving the subsequent thorough cleaning of the sockets.

The procedure is virtually identical to the socket cleaning done when a root canal-treated tooth is removed. It is also important to emphasize that the actual sites of cavitation are usually completely asymptom-

atic and that these sites virtually never "heal" spontaneously. When the larger wisdom tooth extraction
sites are explored months, years, or even decades after
the initial extraction, cavitations are still found nearly
90% of the time (Levy and Huggins, 1996). Sometimes
a larger cavitation needs surgical revision more than
once before a regrowth of new bone completely fills
the defect and eliminates that cavitation as an ongoing
source of toxicity.

Replacement of toxic dental fillings with non-tox-
ic or vastly less toxic substitutes is another way to substantially lessen the daily oxidative stress placed upon
the body's overall antioxidant pool. The best known
and most toxic of these fillings is the mercury-containing amalgam.

However, a majority of other fillings contain
highly toxic chemicals as well, and the body responds
positively to quality antioxidants and other supplementation much more readily when these toxic fillings
have been properly replaced. The replacement of these
fillings needs to be done with the most biocompatible
materials available, and this is best done when guided
by serum biocompatibility testing (Huggins and Levy,
1999).

Similarly, other substances commonly placed in
the mouth are highly toxic and ultimately prooxidant
to nearly all patients. Stainless steel, containing a large
amount of nickel, is still routinely chosen as a base for
crowns. As it costs very little, it is also the most common substance used for braces and partial plates.

Nickel is carcinogenic, and it has been shown to deplete intracellular levels of vitamin C (Salnikow and Kasprzak, 2005). Many other metals frequently used in dental reconstructions in the mouth are also very toxic, and following the results of serum biocompatibility testing to guide the replacement of these materials with less noxious materials is a good way to minimize this significant source of toxicity present in many individuals.

Dental implants are too often a great source of dental toxicity, and sometimes chronic infection, as well. Presently, the routine performance of a dental implant finds the dentist screwing a piece of nickel directly into the bone through an area of evolving cavitation in an area of recent extraction, with significant infection and toxicity already present.

Furthermore, the placement of toxic metal into the bone (versus sitting atop it, as with a crown) appears to often initiate an autoimmune disease process in the body. Such a process rarely relents until the implant is properly removed, in much the same fashion as the removal of the root canal-treated tooth.

The most important first step in getting a Total Dental Revision is to find a dentist who is at least familiar with the above concepts and willing to work with you to get your best results. In order to find such a dentist, call Scientific Health Solutions, Inc. at 800-331-2303 or 719-548-1600 or email at dentists@bestden talmaterials.com. *All referrals:*

Dr Huggins 866-948-4638

This laboratory has worked over the years with a large number of dentists who are familiar with all or most of the procedures noted above, and these dentists use serum biocompatibility testing to try to ensure that other toxic materials are not re-introduced into your mouth. Scientific Health Solutions can help you find a dentist in your area of the United States, as well as in a limited number of other countries around the world.

To recap, dental toxicity is a very large source of prooxidant, vitamin C-neutralizing stress in a large and ever increasing number of individuals today. Avoiding a Total Dental Revision as outlined above while following the other aspects of the anti-atherosclerosis protocol outlined below will eliminate for many individuals the possibility that their atherosclerosis will be reversed.

More likely, only a stabilization or slowing of the atherosclerotic process will be attained by ignoring the Total Dental Revision. However, if you simply cannot bring yourself to follow the suggestions for a Total Dental Revision, your longevity and your general health will still be vastly improved by following the remainder of the protocol. Also, if you cannot do the complete total revision, consider revising the most important parts of dental toxicity, which for most people will be the proper removal of root canal-treated teeth and the proper treatment of chronic periodontal disease.

B. MINIMIZATION OF DIETARY TOXICITY

Unfortunately, eating a healthy diet today is not a simple or even self-obvious matter. Many books on nutrition and diet espouse precisely opposite concepts and suggestions, and virtually all the books have been written by individuals who appear to be eminently qualified to give such advice.

The following advice on proper nutrition comes from my earlier book, *Optimal Nutrition for Optimal Health* (Levy, 2001). However, nearly all of the suggestions for optimal nutrition derive from the dietary interventions that I have repeatedly seen to make chronically sick patients better, and that I have consistently noted to make abnormal blood tests normal, or at least less abnormal, in both sick individuals and in individuals appearing clinically healthy.

Although I advise following all of the recommendations made in the book, here are the most important ones to implement, in a roughly descending order of significance:

- Choose proper food combinations.
- Minimize the intake of high glycemic index foods and refined sugar.
- Chew all foods extremely thoroughly.
- Minimize water and other liquids as drinks with meals.
- Eliminate milk as a beverage.
- Emphasize fresh vegetable intake, but do not be a vegetarian.
- Minimize seafood intake.

Proper food combining is absolutely essential for minimizing the toxicity of the gut. Gut toxicity, especially from poorly digested protein, can be enormous. Anaerobic bacteria, producing toxins with the same level of toxicity as root canals, can predominate in a constipated gut filled with rotting food. A toxic, constipated gut is not unlike a mouth filled with root canals and cavitations. A healthy gut should have a bowel transit time well below 24 hours, meaning that less than one bowel movement per day is a clear sign of heightened bowel toxicity and that your dietary regimen is clearly suboptimal.

High glycemic index foods and refined sugar both promote heart disease. Intake of these items on a regular basis ensures that glucose is always released relatively rapidly into the bloodstream. Glucose directly competes with vitamin C for access into the cells, and minimizing the rate of glucose release into the blood is always highly desirable for optimizing the levels of intracellular vitamin C.

Poor chewing, even though very easily addressed, is a primary reason for less food eventually getting properly digested, and more food ending up rotting and promoting a toxic, constipated gut.

Chewing is incredibly important since the digestive enzymes of the human being are relatively weak and require as much assistance as possible. Animals such as snakes are opposite humans on the digestive spectrum, digesting their food without any chewing at all.

However, in the human, a large portion of food, typically protein, that gets swallowed relatively intact really only has optimal digestion taking place over the outer surface. Chewing not only mixes in the salivary enzymes to get digestion started, it is also essential for substantially increasing and ultimately optimizing the surface area of the food being exposed to the digestive enzymes. It is important to realize that optimizing all of the other digestive factors will never completely compensate for poor chewing at the outset. Poorly chewed food will always result in some degree of a toxic gut.

Water and other liquids with a meal should always be minimized. Quite simply, the body does not have an unlimited supply of enzymes or time to initiate and complete the digestive process.

Particularly in the stomach, in the earlier phases of digestion, it is very important to pay close attention to this advisory. The more water gets mixed in with the food in the stomach, the more dilute the digestive enzymes get, and ultimately the less complete digestion ends up. Also, more dilute stomach contents have a pH that gets closer to neutrality, and the reactive secretion/activation of more digestive enzymes triggered by pH ultimately lessens.

Eliminating milk as a beverage is a very good digestive rule for a number of reasons. Milk is a notoriously bad nutrient to combine with a large number of different foods. Much of the bloating and digestive discomfort that many individuals associate with milk and blame on "lactose intolerance" is really just a reflection of how poorly milk combines with so many different foods.

Milk is also a substantial source of calcium that ultimately promotes the deposition of calcium throughout the body and the blood vessels, strongly supporting and promoting the atherosclerotic process independently. Of course, milk as a liquid should also be avoided for all of the reasons described above with water and the dilution of digestive enzymes.

Fresh vegetables are a very important part of a healthy diet. However, avoiding meat completely is rarely good for anybody. A regular source of cholesterol is essential for coping with and helping to neutralize the daily toxin exposures that are faced by all. Of course, meat needs to be digested properly or it can ultimately be a significant source of bacterial toxicity rather than optimal nutrition. Fresh vegetables are also a primary source of dietary vitamin C and other important antioxidants.

Seafood contains greater amounts of mercury than any other food source. Overall, the less seafood you consume, the better off you are because of this direct assault on your overall antioxidant status. Pregnant women should have no seafood in their diets at all. However, all individuals interested in minimizing their daily toxin exposures should minimize their intakes of seafood as well.

C. RECOMMENDED SUPPLEMENTATION

The following supplementation regimen is recommended in concert with the measures outlined above and based on the concepts presented in this book for minimizing overall daily net toxin exposure and for optimizing the ability of the artery to regenerate itself and reverse any existing atherosclerosis. These supplements are presented very roughly in order of descending priority. They all are very important for the health of the blood vessel, and the typical diet does not even come close to supplying enough of these essential vitamins, minerals, and nutrients.

- L-ascorbic acid (vitamin C): 3,000 to 9,000 mg daily
- L-lysine: 3,000 to 6,000 mg daily
- L-proline: 500 to 1,500 mg daily
- L-arginine: 500 to 1,500 mg daily
- Magnesium glycinate (or other magnesium-amino acid chelate): 200 to 1,000 mg daily
- Menatetrenone (vitamin K2): 3 to 9 mg daily
- Cholecalciferol (vitamin D3): 400 to 1,000 IU daily
- Mixed tocopherols (vitamin E source): 400 to 1,000 IU daily
- Beta carotene (vitamin A source): 25,000 to 50,000 IU daily
- L-carnosine: 200 to 1,000 mg daily
- Omega-3 (n-3) fatty acids: 1,000 mg to 3,000 mg daily
- Thiamine (vitamin B1): 50 to 500 mg daily

- Pyridoxine (vitamin B6): 25 to 100 mg daily
- Riboflavin (vitamin B2): 5 to 15 mg daily
- Pantothenic acid (vitamin B5) 10 to 15 mg daily
- Biotin (vitamin B7): 300 to 500 micrograms daily
- Folic acid (vitamin B9): 400 to 500 micrograms daily
- Cobalamin (vitamin B12): 15 to 20 micrograms daily
- Niacin (vitamin B3): 20 to 25 mg daily
- Coenzyme Q10: 50 to 250 mg daily
- Superoxide dismutase (SOD): 100 to 400 mg daily
- Chondroitin sulfate C (chondroitin 6-sulfate): 500 to 1,500 mg daily
- Methylsulfonylmethane (MSM): 500 to 1,500 mg daily
- Glucosamine: 500 to 1,500 mg daily
- Glutathione: 500 to 1,500 mg daily
- N-acetylcysteine: 500 to 1,500 mg daily
- Chromium: 100 to 200 micrograms daily
- Manganese: 0.5 to 1.0 mg daily
- Zinc: 10 to 20 mg daily
- Selenium: 100 to 200 micrograms daily
- Vanadium: 10 to 50 micrograms daily
- Indium: 25 to 50 micrograms daily
- Boron: 15 to 25 micrograms daily

Note that the above recommendations do not include calcium. Much of the atherosclerosis "epidemic" seen today is strongly fueled by the indiscriminate supplementation of calcium. Osteoporosis is readily treated effectively with the regimen as noted above, and with the exception of rare metabolic disorders, the supplementation of calcium is never recommended.

These recommendations for the prevention and reversal of atherosclerosis are based on the scientific evidence as already presented in this book. Of course, the diversity of biology dictates that everyone who follows the above regimen will not have their heavily diseased arteries revert to normal in appearance and physiology. However, many, if not a vast majority, should have exactly that dramatic a response if all aspects of the protocol are followed.

For those who simply cannot or will not follow the recommendation for a Total Dental Revision, the rest of the protocol should still improve overall health dramatically. Atherosclerosis should still be slowed in its progression, and in those individuals who have lesser amounts of dental toxicity, probably reversed as well.

Rath and Niedzwiecki (1996) already showed that a less comprehensive protocol involving only supplementation could reliably lessen the natural progression rate of coronary artery calcification. They also documented in individual cases the reversal and complete resolution of previously existing coronary artery calcification.

This spectrum of results achieved further supports the need for minimizing daily toxin exposure as an essential element of reversing atherosclerosis. The

patients with the least daily toxin exposure undoubtedly were the best responders to the Rath and Niedzwiecki protocol, although this was not specifically analyzed. I would encourage all readers of this book who
undergo all or part of the suggested protocol outlined
above to let me know how they do clinically (chest
pain) and objectively (angiograms, stress tests, ECHO-
cardiograms, and/or coronary artery calcium scores)
at "drlevy@tomlevymd.com".

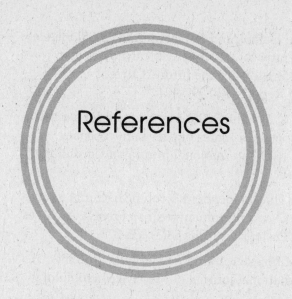

References

Abbasy, M. (1937) XLIX. The diuretic action of vitamin C. The Biochemical Journal 31:339-342.

Abt, A., S. von Schuching, and J. Roe (1959) Connective tissue studies. II. The effect of vitamin C deficiency on healed wounds. Bulletin of the Johns Hopkins Hospital 105:67-76.

Adam, E., J. Melnick, J. Probtsfield, B. Petrie, J. Burek, K. Bailey, C. McCollum, and M. DeBakey (1987) High levels of cytomegalovirus antibody in patients requiring vascular surgery for atherosclerosis. Lancet 2(8554):291-293.

Adams, C. and R. Morgan (1967) The effect of saturated and polyunsaturated lecithins on the resorption of 4-14C-cholesterol from subcutaneous implants. Journal of Pathology and Bacteriology 94(1):73-76.

Adams, C., Y. Abdulla, O. Bayliss, and R. Morgan (1967) Modification of aortic atheroma and fatty liver in saturated and polyunsaturated lecithins. Journal of Pathology and Bacteriology 94(1):77-87.

Aleo, J. (1981) Diabetes and periodontal disease. Possible role of vitamin C deficiency: an hypothesis. Journal of Periodontology 52(5):251-254.

Aljaroudi, W., A. Halabi, and R. Harrington (2005) Platelet inhibitor therapy for patients with cardiovascular disease: looking toward the future. Current Hematology Reports 4(5):397-404.

Allison, M, and C. Wright (2005) Age and gender are the strongest clinical correlates of prevalent coronary calcification (R1). International Journal of Cardiology 98(2):325-330.

Alouf, J. (1981) [Thiol-dependent cytolytic bacterial toxins: streptolysin O and prominent toxins]. French. Archives de l'Institut Pasteur de Tunis 58(3):355-373.

Alouf, J. (2000) Cholesterol-binding cytolytic protein toxins. International Journal of Medical Microbiology 290(4-5):351-356.

Altman, R., G. Schaeffer, C. Salles, A. Ramos de Souza, and P. Cotias (1980) Phospholipids associated with vitamin C in experimental atherosclerosis. Arzneimittelforschung 30(4):627-630.

Anitschkow, N. (1928) Uber die ruckbildungsvorgange bei der experimentellen atherosklerose. Verhandl d deutsch path Gesellsch 23:473-478.

Anitschkow, N. (1933) Experimental arteriosclerosis in animals. In: Cowdry, E. (ed) Arteriosclerosis: A Survey of the Problem. New York, NY: The Macmillan Company.

Appels, A., C. Jenkins, and R. Rosenman (1982) Coronary-prone behavior in the Netherlands: a cross-cultural validation study. Journal of Behavioral Medicine 5(1): 83-90.

Appels, A., P. Mulder, M. van't Hof, C. Jenkins, J. van Houtem, and F. Tan (1987) A prospective study of the Jenkins Activity Survey as a risk indicator for coronary heart disease in the Netherlands. Journal of Chronic Diseases 40(10):959-965.

Archer, S., K. Liu, A. Dyer, K. Ruth, D. Jacobs, Jr., L. van Horn, J. Hilner, and P. Savage (1998) Relationship between changes in dietary sucrose and high density lipoprotein cholesterol: the CARDIA study. Coronary Artery Risk Development in Young Adults. Annals of Epidemiology 8(7):433-438.

Ariyo, A., M. Haan, C. Tangen, J. Rutledge, M. Cushman, A. Dobs, and C. Furberg (2000) Depressive symptoms and risks of coronary heart disease and mortality in elderly Americans. Cardiovascular Health Study Collaborative Research Group. Circulation 102(15): 1773-1779.

Arntz, H., S. Willich, C. Schreiber, T. Bruggemann, R. Stern, and H. Schultheiss (2000) Diurnal, weekly and seasonal variation of sudden death. Population-based analysis of 24,061 consecutive cases. European Heart Journal 21(4):259-261.

Austin, M., M. King, K. Vranizan, and R. Krauss (1990) Atherogenic lipoprotein phenotype. A proposed genetic marker for coronary heart disease risk. Circulation 82(2):495-506.

Babu, J., S. Sundravel, G. Arumugam, R. Renuka, N. Deepa, and P. Sachdanandam (2000) Salubrious effect of vitamin C and vitamin E on tamoxifen-treated women in breast cancer with reference to plasma lipid and lipoprotein levels. Cancer Letters 151(1):1-5.

Bailey, C. (1917) Arteriosclerosis and glomerulonephritis. Journal of Experimental Medicine 25:109.

Baker, L. (1929) Journal of Experimental Medicine 49:163.

Banerjee, S. (1943) Vitamin C and carbohydrate metabolism. Nature 152(3855):329.

Banerjee, S. (1944) Relation to scurvy to histological changes in the pancreas. Nature 153(3881):344-345.

Banerjee, S. and N. Ghosh (1947) Relation of scurvy to glucose tolerance test, liver glycogen, and insulin content of pancreas of guinea pigs. Journal of Biological Chemistry 168:207-211.

Banerjee, S. and H. Singh (1958) Cholesterol metabolism in scorbutic guinea pigs. Journal of Biological Chemistry 233(1):336-339.

Banerjee, S. and A. Bandyopadhyay (1963) Plasma lipids in scurvy: effect of ascorbic acid supplement and insulin treatment. Proceedings of the Society for Experimental Biology and Medicine 112:372-374.

Barnes, M. (1969) Ascorbic acid and the biosynthesis of collagen and elastin. Bibliotheca Nutritio et Dieta 13: 86-98.

Bates, C., C. Walmsley, A. Prentice, and S. Finch (1998) Does vitamin C reduce blood pressure? Results of a large study of people aged 65 or older. Journal of Hypertension 16(7):925-932.

Baynes, J. (1991) Role of oxidative stress in development of complications in diabetes. Diabetes 40(4):405-412.

Beck, J., J. Pankow, H. Tyroler, and S. Offenbacher (1999) Dental infections and atherosclerosis. American Heart Journal 138(5 Pt 2):S528-533.

Becker, A., O. de Boer, and A. van der Wal (2001) The role of inflammation and infection in coronary heart disease. Annual Review of Medicine 52:289-297.

Beetens, J., M. Coene, A. Verheyen, L. Zonnekeyn, and A. Herman (1984) Influence of vitamin C on the metabolism of arachidonic acid and the development of aortic lesions during experimental atherosclerosis in rabbits. Biomedica Biochimica Acta 43(8-9):S273-S276.

Belting, C., J. Hinkler, and C. Dummett (1964) Influence of diabetes mellitus on the severity of periodontal disease. Journal of Periodontology 35:476.

Bensley, S. (1934) On the presence, properties and distribution of the intercellular ground substance of loose connective tissue. The Anatomical Record 60:93-109.

Berenson, G. (1961) Studies of "ground substance" of the vessel wall and alterations in atherosclerosis and related diseases. Journal of Atherosclerosis Research 1: 386-393.

Bielak, L., G. Klee, P. Sheedy, S. Turner, R. Schwartz, and P. Peyser (2000) Association of fibrinogen with quantity of coronary artery calcification measured by electron beam computed tomography. Arteriosclerosis, Thrombosis, and Vascular Biology 20(9):2167-2171.

Bielicki, J., M. McCall, J. van den Berg, F. Kuypers, and T. Forte (1995) Copper and gas-phase cigarette smoke inhibit plasma lecithin:cholesterol acyltransferase activity by different mechanisms. Journal of Lipid Research 36(2):322-331.

Bigley, R., M. Wirth, D. Layman, M. Riddle, and L. Stankova (1983) Interaction between glucose and dehydroascorbate transport in human neutrophils and fibroblasts. Diabetes 32(6):545-548.

Bishop, N., C. Schorah, and J. Wales (1985) The effect of vitamin C supplementation on diabetic hyperlipidaemia: a double blind, crossover study. Diabetic Medicine: A Journal of the British Diabetic Association 2(2):121-124.

Blake-Mortimer, J., A. Winefield, and A. Chalmers (1998) The effect of depression in an animal model on 5'-ectonucleotidase, antibody production, and tissue ascorbate stores. The Journal of General Psychology 125(2):129-146.

Blanck, T. and B. Peterkofsky (1975) The stimulation of collagen secretion by ascorbate as a result of increased proline hydroxylation in chick embryo fibroblasts. Archives of Biochemistry and Biophysics 171(1):259-267.

Bloomer, A., S. Nash, H. Price, and R. Welch (1977) A study of pesticide residues in Michigan's general population, 1968-70. Pesticides Monitoring Journal 11(3):111-115.

Blum, A., V. Hadas, M. Burke, I. Yust, and A. Kessler (2005) Viral load of the human immunodeficiency virus could be an independent risk factor for endothelial dysfunction. Clinical Cardiology 28(3):149-153.

Bobek, P., E. Ginter, L. Ozdin, and L. Mikus (1980) The effect of chronic marginal vitamin C deficiency on the rate of secretion and the removal of plasma triglycerides in guinea-pigs. Physiologia Bohemoslovaca 29(4):337-343.

Boers, G. (2000) Mild hyperhomocysteinemia is an independent risk factor of arterial vascular disease. Seminars in Thrombosis and Hemostasis 26(3):291-295.

Booker, W., F. DaCosta, W. Jones, C. Froix, and E. Robinson (1957) Cholesterol-ascorbic acid relationship; changes in plasma and cell ascorbic acid and plasma cholesterol following administration of ascorbic acid and cholesterol. American Journal of Physiology 189:75-77.

Boonmark, N., X. Lou, Z. Yang, K. Schwartz, J. Zhang, E. Rubin, and R. Lawn (1997) Modification of apolipoprotein(a) lysine binding site reduces atherosclerosis in transgenic mice. Journal of Clinical Investigation 100(3):558-564.

Boos, C. and G. Lip (2006) Blood clotting, inflammation, and thrombosis in cardiovascular events: perspectives. Frontiers in Bioscience: a Journal and Virtual Library 11:328-336.

Bordia, A., D. Paliwal, K. Jain, and L. Kothari (1978) Acute effect of ascorbic acid on fibrinolytic activity. Atherosclerosis 30(4):351-354.

Boskey, A., R. Blank, and S. Doty (2001) Vitamin C-sulfate inhibits mineralization in chondrocyte cultures: a caveat. Matrix Biology: Journal of the International Society for Matrix Biology 20(2):99-106.

Bostom, A., L. Yanek, A. Hume, C. Eaton, W. McQuade, M. Nadeau, G. Perrone, P. Jacques, and J. Selhub (1994) High dose ascorbate supplementation fails to affect plasma homocyst(e)ine levels in patients with coronary heart disease. Atherosclerosis 111(2):267-270.

Bothwell, T., B. Bradlow, P. Jacobs, K. Keeley, S. Kramer, H. Seftel, and S Zail (1964) Iron metabolism in scurvy with special reference to erythropoiesis. British Journal of Haematology 10:50.

Boumans, P. and P. Mier (1970) Cutaneous acid mucopolysaccharides in ascorbic acid deficiency. Dermatologica 141(3):234-238.

Bourne, G. (1942) Vitamin C and repair of injured tissues. Lancet 2:661-664.

Bourquin, A. and E. Musmanno (1953) Preliminary report on the effect of smoking on the ascorbic acid content of whole blood. American Journal of Digestive Diseases 20:75-77.

Boushey, C., S. Beresford, G. Omenn, and A. Motulsky (1995) A quantitative assessment of plasma homocysteine as a risk factor for vascular disease. Probable benefits of increasing folic acid intakes. Journal of the American Medical Association 274(13): 1049-1057.

Brophy, J., P. Brassard, and C. Bourgault (2005) The benefit of cholesterol-lowering medications after coronary revascularization: a population study. American Heart Journal 150(2):282-286.

Brown, B., J. Albers, L. Fisher, S. Schaefer, J. Lin, C. Kaplan, X. Zhao, B. Risson, V. Fitzpatrick, and H. Dodge (1990) Regression of coronary artery disease as a result of intensive lipid-lowering therapy in men with high levels of apolipoprotein B. The New England Journal of Medicine 323(19):1289-1298.

Brown, B., X. Zhao, D. Sacco, and J. Albers (1993) Arteriographic view of treatment to achieve regression of coronary atherosclerosis and to prevent plaque disruption and clinical cardiovascular events. British Heart Journal 69(1 Suppl):S48-S53.

Brown, B., X. Zhao, D. Sacco, and J. Albers (1993a) Atherosclerosis regression, plaque disruption, and cardiovascular events: a rationale for lipid lowering in coronary artery disease. Annual Review of Medicine 44:365-376.

Brown, B., X. Zhao, D. Sacco, and J. Albers (1993b) Lipid lowering and plaque regression. New insights into prevention of plaque disruption and clinical events in coronary disease. Circulation 87(6):1781-1791.

Brown, D., W. Giles, and J. Croft (2001) White blood cell count: an independent predictor of coronary heart disease mortality among a national cohort. Journal of Clinical Epidemiology 54(3):316-322.

Brown, M. and J. Goldstein (1983) Lipoprotein metabolism in the macrophage: implications for cholesteroldeposition in atherosclerosis. Annual Review of Biochemistry 52:223-261.

Brown, M. and J. Goldstein (1987) Plasma lipoproteins: teaching old dogmas new tricks. Nature 330(6144):113-114.

Buchwald, H., R. Varco, J. Matts, J. Long, L. Fitch, G. Campbell, M. Pearce, A. Yellin, W. Edmiston, R. Smink, Jr. et al. (1990) Effect of partial ileal bypass on mortality and morbidity from coronary heart disease in patients with hypercholesterolemia. Report of the Program on the Surgical Control of Hyperlipidemias (POSCH). The New England Journal of Medicine 323(14):946-955.

Buddecke, E. (1962) Chemical changes in the ground substance of the vessel wall in arteriosclerosis. Journal of Atherosclerosis Research 2:32-46.

Buffon, A., G. Liuzzo, L. Biasucci, P. Pasqualetti, V. Ramazzotti, A. Rebuzzi, F. Crea, and A. Maseri (1999) Preprocedural serum levels of C-reactive protein predict early complications and late restenosis after coronary angioplasty. Journal of the American College of Cardiology 34(5):1512-1521.

Bunout, D., A. Garrido, M. Suazo, R. Kauffman, P. Venegas, P. de la Maza, M. Petermann, and S. Hirsch (2000) Effects of supplementation with folic acid and antioxidant vitamins on homocysteine levels and LDL oxidation in coronary patients. Nutrition 16(2):107-110.

Burke, A., P. Varghese, E. Peterson, G. Malcolm, A. Farb, and R. Virmani (2001) Large lipid core and extensive plaque burden are features of coronary atherosclerosis in patients with non-insulin dependent diabetes mellitus. Journal of the American College of Cardiology 37(2 Supp A):257A.

Burkhardt, D. and P. Ghosh (1987) Laboratory evaluation of antiarthritic drugs as potential chondroprotective agents. Seminars in Arthritis and Rheumatism 17(2 Suppl 1):3-34.

Cameron, E. (1976) Biological function of ascorbic acid and the pathogenesis of scurvy: a working hypothesis. Medical Hypotheses 2(4):154-163.

Cantin, B., D. Zhu, P. Wen, S. Panchal, J. Gwathmey, G. Reaven, and H. Valantine (2002) Preferential involvement of larger vessels in a rat model of diabetes-induced graft vasculopathy. The Journal of Heart and Lung Transplantation: the Official Publication of the International Society for Heart Transplantation 21(9):1040-1043.

Capuano, V., N. Lamaida, M. De Martino, and G. Mazzotta (1995) Association between white blood cell count and risk factors of coronary artery disease. Giornale Italiano di Cardiologia 25(9):1145-1152.

Carlson, L., M. Danielson, I. Ekberg, B. Klintemar, and G. Rosenhamer (1977) Reduction of myocardial reinfarction by the combined treatment with clofibrate and nicotinic acid. Atherosclerosis 28(1):81-86.

Carlson, L. and L. Bottiger (1985) Risk factors for ischaemic heart disease in men and women. Results of the 19-year follow-up of the Stockholm Prospective Study. Acta Medica Scandinavica 218(2):207-211.

Carney, R., K. Freedland, R. Veith, and A. Jaffe (1999) Can treating depression reduce mortality after an acute myocardial infarction? Psychosomatic Medicine 61(5): 666-675.

Carr, A., B. Zhu, and B. Frei (2000) Potential antiatherogenic mechanisms of ascorbate (vitamin C) and α-tocopherol (vitamin E). Circulation Research 87(5):349-354.

Cassidy, A., L. Bielak, Y. Zhou, P. Sheedy, S. Turner, J. Breen, P. Araoz, I. Kullo, X. Lin, and P. Peyser (2005) Progression of subclinical coronary atherosclerosis: does obesity make a difference? Circulation 111(15): 1877-1882.

Cecil Textbook of Medicine (2000) 21st edition. Edited by Goldman, L. and J. Bennett. Philadelphia, PA: W.B. Saunders Company.

Chambers, J., A. McGregor, J. Jean-Marie, O. Obeid, and J. Kooner (1999) Demonstration of rapid onset vascular endothelial dysfunction after hyperhomocysteinemia. An effect reversible with vitamin C therapy. Circulation 99(9):1156-1160.

Chamiec, T., K. Herbaczynska-Cedro, and L. Ceremuzynski (1996) Effects of antioxidant vitamins C and E on signal-averaged electrocardiogram in acute myocardial infarction. The American Journal of Cardiology 77(4):237-241.

Chatterjee, I., S. Gupta, A. Majumder, B. Nandi, and N. Subramanian (1975) Effect of ascorbic acid on histamine metabolism in scorbutic guinea-pigs. Journal of Physiology 251(2):271-279.

Chen, C. and G. Loo (1995) Effect of peroxyl radicals on lecithin/cholesterol acyltransferase activity in human plasma. Lipids 30(7):627-631.

Chen, M., M. Hutchinson, R. Pecoraro, W. Lee, and F. Labbe (1983) Hyperglycemia-induced intracellular depletion of ascorbic acid in human mononuclear leukocytes. Diabetes 32(11):1078-1081.

Cheng, T. (2000) Why is atherosclerosis non-existent in human intramyocardial coronary arteries? Atherosclerosis 153(1):259.

Cheraskin, E., W. Ringsdorf, Jr., and B. Hicks (1974) Daily vitamin C consumption and reported cardiovascular findings. Journal of the International Academy of Preventive Medicine 1(1):31-44.

Chi, M., M. El-Halawani, P. Waibel, and C. Mirocha (1981) Effects of T-2 toxin on brain catecholamines and selected blood components in growing chickens. Poultry Science 60(1):137-141.

Clark, E. and E. Clark (1918) On the reaction of certain cells in the tadpole's tail toward vital dyes. The Anatomical Record 15:151.

Clark, E. and E. Clark (1933) Further observations on living lymphatic vessels in the transparent chamber in the rabbit's ear—their relation to the tissue spaces. American Journal of Anatomy 52:273-305.

Clarke, R., L. Daly, K. Robinson, E. Naughten, S. Cahalane, B. Fowler, and I. Graham (1991) Hyperhomocysteinemia: an independent risk factor for vascular disease. The New England Journal of Medicine 324(17):1149-1155.

Clejan, S., S. Japa, C. Clemetson, S. Hasabnis, O. David, and J. Talano (2002) Blood histamine is associated with coronary artery disease, cardiac events and severity of inflammation and atherosclerosis. Journal of Cellular and Molecular Medicine 6(4):583-592.

Clemetson, C. (1980) Histamine and ascorbic acid in human blood. The Journal of Nutrition 110(4):662-668.

Clemetson, C. (1999) The key role of histamine in the development of atherosclerosis and coronary heart disease. Medical Hypotheses 52(1):1-8.

Cocchi, P., M. Silenzi, G. Calabri, and G. Salvi (1980) Antidepressant effect of vitamin C. Pediatrics 65(4):862-863.

Cohen, H., S. Madhavan, and M. Alderman (2001) History of treatment for depression: risk factor for myocardial infarction in hypertensive patients. Psychosomatic Medicine 63(2):203-209.

Cohen, J., S. Syme, C. Jenkins, A. Kagan, and S. Zyzanski (1979) Cultural context of type A behavior and risk for CHD: a study of Japanese American males. Journal of Behavioral Medicine 2(4):375-384.

Cohen, M. (1955) The effect of large doses of ascorbic acid on gingival tissue at puberty. Journal of Dental Research 34(Abstract):750.

Cooper, A. and A. Heagerty (1998) Endothelial dysfunction in human intramyocardial small arteries in atherosclerosis and hypercholesterolemia. The American Journal of Physiology 275(4 Pt 2):H1482-H1488.

Coronary Drug Project Research Group (1975) Clofibrate and niacin in coronary heart disease. Journal of the American Medical Association 231(4):360-381.

Corti, R., R. Hutter, J. Badimon, and V. Fuster (2004) Evolving concepts in the triad of atherosclerosis, inflammation and thrombosis. Journal of Thrombosis and Thrombolysis 17(1):35-44.

Correia, M. and W. Haynes (2004) Leptin, obesity and cardiovascular disease. Current Opinion in Nephrology and Hypertension 13(2):215-223.

Cowan, L., D. O'Connell, M. Criqui, E. Barrett-Connor, T. Bush, and R. Wallace (1990) Cancer mortality and lipid and lipoprotein levels. Lipid Research Clinics Program Mortality Follow-up Study. American Journal of Epidemiology 131(3):468-482.

Crawford, T. and C. Levene (1953) Medial thinning in atheroma. Journal of Pathology and Bacteriology 66: 19-23.

Cunningham, J. (1998) The glucose/insulin system and vitamin C: implications in insulin-dependent diabetes mellitus. Journal of the American College of Nutrition 17(2):105-108.

Cunningham, M. and R. Pasternak (1988) The potential role of viruses in the pathogenesis of atherosclerosis. Circulation 77(5):964-966.

Cushing, G., J. Gaubatz, M. Nava, B. Burdick, T. Bocan, J. Guyton, D. Weilbaecher, M. DeBakey, G. Lawrie, and J. Morrisett (1989) Quantitation and localization of apolipoproteins(a) and B in coronary artery bypass vein grafts resected at re-operation. Arteriosclerosis 9(5):593-603.

de Leeuw, K., C. Kallenberg, and M. Bijl (2005) Accelerated atherosclerosis in patients with systemic autoimmune diseases. Annals of the New York Academy of Sciences 1051:362-371.

den Heijer, M., T. Koster, H. Blom, G. Bos, E. Briet, P. Reitsma, J. Vandenbroucke, and R. Rosendaal (1996) Hyperhomocysteinemia as a risk factor for deep-vein thrombosis. The New England Journal of Medicine 334(12):759-762.

Dahl-Jorgensen, K., J. Larsen, and K. Hanssen (2005) Atherosclerosis in childhood and adolescent type I diabetes: early disease, early treatment? Diabetologia 48(8):1445-1453.

Dandona, P., A. Aljada, P. Mohanty, H. Ghanim, W. Hamouda, E. Assian, and S. Ahmad (2001) Insulin inhibits intranuclear nuclear factor kappaB and stimulates IkappaB in mononuclear cells in obese subjects: evidence for an anti-inflammatory effect? The Journal of Clinical Endocrinology and Metabolism 86(7):3257-3265.

Datey, K., C. Dalvi, N. Mehta, and N. Purandare (1968) Ascorbic acid and experimental atherosclerosis. Journal of the Association of Physicians of India 16(9):567-570.

Day, C., J. Powell, and R. Levy (1975) Sulfated polysaccharide inhibition of aortic uptake of low density lipoproteins. Artery 1(2):126-137.

DeForrest, J. and T. Hollis (1980) Relationship between low intensity shear stress, aortic histamine formation, and aortic albumin uptake. Experimental and Molecular Pathology 32(3):217-225.

Dent, F., R. Hayes, and W. Booker (1951) Further evidence of cholesterol-ascorbic acid antagonism in blood; role of adrenocortical hormones. Federation Proceedings 18:291.

Diaz-Araya, G., D. Nettle, P. Castro, F. Miranda, D. Greig, X. Campos, M. Chiong, C. Nazzal, R. Corbalan, and S. Lavandero (2002) Oxidative stress after reperfusion with primary coronary angioplasty: lack of effect of glucose-insulin-potassium infusion. Critical Care Medicine 30(2):417-421.

Dingchao, H., Q. Zhiduan, H. Liye, and F. Xiaodong (1994) The protective effects of high-dose ascorbic acid on myocardium against reperfusion injury during and after cardiopulmonary bypass. The Thoracic and Cardiovascular Surgeon 42(5):276-278.

Dobiasova, M. (1983) Lecithin:cholesterol acyltransferase and the regulation of endogenous cholesterol transport. Advances in Lipid Research 20:107-194.

Dobson, H., M. Muir, and R. Hume (1984) The effect of ascorbic acid on the seasonal variations in serum cholesterol levels. Scottish Medical Journal 29(3):176-182.

Dodds, M. (1969) Sex as a factor in blood levels of ascorbic acid. Journal of the American Dietetic Association 54(1):32-33.

Dorja, A., Y. Sherer, P. Meroni, and Y. Shoenfeld (2005) Inflammation and accelerated atherosclerosis: basic mechanisms. Rheumatic Diseases Clinics of North America 31(2):355-362, viii.

Dorr, A., K. Gundersen, J. Schneider, Jr., T. Spencer, and W. Martin (1978) Colestipol hydrochloride in hypercholesterolemic patients-effect on serum cholesterol and mortality. Journal of Chronic Disease 31(1):5-14.

Dou, C., D. Xu, and W. Wells (1997) Studies on the essential role of ascorbic acid in the energy dependent release of insulin from pancreatic islets. Biochemical and Biophysical Research Communications 231(3):820-822.

Douglas, A., M. Dunnigan, T. Allan, and J. Rawles (1995) Seasonal variation in coronary heart disease in Scotland. Journal of Epidemiology and Community Health 49(6):575-582.

Drzewoski, J., L. Czupryniak, G. Chwatko, and E. Bald (2000) Hyperhomocysteinemia in poorly controlled type 2 diabetes patients. Diabetes, Nutrition & Metabolism 13(6):319-324.

Duff, G. (1935) Experimental cholesterol arteriosclerosis and its relationship to human arteriosclerosis. Archives of Pathology 20:81-123, 259-304.

Duffy, S., N. Gokce, M. Holbrook, A. Huang, B. Frei, J. Keaney, and J. Vita (1999) Treatment of hypertension with ascorbic acid. Lancet 354(9195):2048-2049.

Dufty, W. (1975) Sugar Blues. New York, NY: Warner Books, Inc.

Durand, C., M. Audinot, and S. Frajdenrajch (1962) Hypovitaminose C latente et tabac. Concours Medical 84:4801.

Dusinovic, S., D. Mijalkovic, Z. Saicic, J. Duric, Z. Zunic, V. Niketic, and M. Spasic (1998) Antioxidative defense in human myocardial reperfusion injury. Journal of Environmental Pathology, Toxicology and Oncology 17(3-4):281-284.

Edward, M. and R. Oliver (1983) Changes in the synthesis, distribution and sulphation of glycosaminoglycans of cultured human skin fibroblasts upon ascorbate feeding. Journal of Cell Science 64:245-254.

Emingil, G., E. Buduneli, A. Aliyev, A. Akilli, and G. Atilla (2000) Association between periodontal disease and acute myocardial infarction. Journal of Periodontology 71(12):1882-1886.

Engel, U. (1971) Glycosaminoglycans in the aorta of six animal species. A chemical and morphological comparison of their topographical distribution. Atherosclerosis 13(1):45-60.

Enquselassie, F., A. Dobson, H. Alexander, and P. Steele (1993) Seasons, temperature and coronary disease. International Journal of Epidemiology 22(4):632-636.

Ensrud, K. and R. Grimm (1992) The white blood cell count and risk for coronary heart disease. American Heart Journal 124(1):207-213.

Enstrom, J., L. Kanim, and M. Klein (1992) Vitamin C intake and mortality among a sample of the United States population. Epidemiology 3(3):194-202.

Erden, F., S. Gulenc, M. Torun, Z. Kocer, B. Simsek, and S. Nebioglu (1985) Ascorbic acid effect on some lipid fractions in human beings. Acta Vitaminologica et Enzymologica 7(1-2):131-137.

Eryol, N., H. Kilic, A. Gul, I. Ozdogru, T. Inanc, A. Dogan, R. Topsakal, and E. Basar (2005) Are the high levels of cytomegalovirus antibodies a determinant in the development of coronary artery disease? International Heart Journal 46(2):205-209.

Evans, R., L. Currie, and A. Campbell (1982) The distribution of ascorbic acid between various cellular components of blood, in normal individuals, and its relation to the plasma concentration. British Journal of Nutrition 47(3):473-482.

Fabricant, C., J. Fabricant, M. Litrenta, and C. Minick (1978) Virus-induced atherosclerosis. Journal of Experimental Medicine 148(1):335-340.

Fabricant, C., J. Fabricant, C. Minick, and M. Litrenta (1983) Herpesvirus-induced atherosclerosis in chickens. Federation Proceedings 42(8):2476-2479.

Falch, J., M. Mowe, and T. Bohmer (1998) Low levels of serum ascorbic acid in elderly patients with hip fracture. Scandinavian Journal of Clinical Laboratory Investigation 58(3):225-228.

Fehily, A., J. Yarnell, P. Sweetnam, and P. Elwood (1993) Diet and incident ischaemic heart disease: the Caerphilly Study. The British Journal of Nutrition 69(2): 303-314.

Ferketich, A., J. Schwartzbaum, D. Frid, and M. Moeschberger (2000) Depression as an antecedent to heart disease among women and men in the NHANES I study. National Health and Nutrition Examination Survey. Archives of Internal Medicine 160(9):1261-1268.

Figueiredo, P., C. Catani, and T. Yano (2003) Serum high-density lipoprotein (HDL) inhibits in vitro enterohemolysin (EHly) activity produced by enteropathogenic Escherichia coli. FEMS Immunology and Medical Microbiology 38(1):53-57.

Finamore, F., R. Feldman, and G. Cosgrove (1976) L-ascorbic acid, L-ascorbate 2-sulfate, and atherogenesis. International Journal for Vitamin and Nutrition Research 46(3):275-285.

Fishbaine, B. and G. Butterfield (1984) Ascorbic acid status of running and sedentary men. International Journal for Vitamin and Nutrition Research 54(2-3):273.

Fisher, D., A. Markitziu, D. Fishel, and L. Brayer (1984) A 4 year follow-up study of alveolar bone height influenced by two dissimilar Class II amalgam restorations. Journal of Oral Rehabilitation 11(4):399-405.

Fisher, E., S. McLennan, H. Tada, S. Heffernan, D. Yue, and J. Turtle (1991) Interaction of ascorbic acid and glucose on production of collagen and proteoglycan by fibroblasts. Diabetes 40(3):371-376.

Ford, E. and S. Liu (2001) Glycemic index and serum high-density lipoprotein cholesterol concentration among US adults. Archives of Internal Medicine 161(4):572-576.

Foster-Powell, K. and J. Miller (1995) International tables of glycemic index. The American Journal of Clinical Nutrition 62(4):871S-890S.

Fotherby, M., J. Williams, L. Forster, P. Craner, and G. Ferns (2000) Effect of vitamin C on ambulatory blood pressure and plasma lipids in older persons. Journal of Hypertension 18(4):411-415.

Frank, E. (1993) Benefits of stopping smoking. The Western Journal of Medicine 159(1):83-86.

Franz, W., G. Sands, and H. Heyl (1956) Blood ascorbic acid level in bioflavonoid and ascorbic acid therapy of common cold. Journal of the American Medical Association 162:1224.

Frei, B. (1999) On the role of vitamin C and other antioxidants in atherogenesis and vascular dysfunction. Proceedings of the Society for Experimental Biology and Medicine. Society for Experimental Biology and Medicine (New York, N.Y.) 222(3):196-204.

Frei, B., R. Stocker, L. England, and B. Ames (1990) Ascorbate: the most effective antioxidant in human blood plasma. Advances in Experimental Medicine and Biology 264:155-163.

Frick, M., O. Elo, K. Haapa, O. Heinonen, P. Heinsalmi, P. Helo, J. Huttunen, P. Kaitaniemi, P. Koskinen, V. Manninen, et al. (1987) Helsinki Heart Study: primary-prevention with gemfibrozil in middle-aged men with dyslipemia. The New England Journal of Medicine 317(20):1237-1245.

Frostegard, J. (2005) Atherosclerosis in patients with autoimmune disorders. Arteriosclerosis, Thrombosis, and Vascular Biology 25(9):1776-1785.

Gackowski, D., M. Kruszewski, A. Jawien, M. Ciecierski, and R. Olinski (2001) Further evidence that oxidative stress may be a risk factor responsible for the development of atherosclerosis. Free Radical Biology & Medicine 31(4):542-547.

Galley, H., J. Thornton, P. Howdle, B. Walker, and N. Webster (1997) Combination oral antioxidant supplementation reduces blood pressure. Clinical Science 92(4):361-365.

Gamble, J., P. Grewal, and I. Gartside (2000) Vitamin C modifies the cardiovascular and microvascular responses to cigarette smoke inhalation in man. Clinical Science 98(4):455-460.

Gerhardsson, M., U. Rosenqvist, A. Ahlbom, and L. Carlson (1986) Serum cholesterol and cancer—a retrospective case-control study. International Journal of Epidemiology 15(2):155-159.

Gero, S., T. Gergely, L. Devenyi, et al. (1961) Role of intimal mucoid substances in the pathogenesis of atherosclerosis. I. Complex formation in vitro between mucopolysaccharides from atherosclerotic aortic intimas and plasma β-lipoprotein and fibrinogen. Journal of Atherosclerosis Research 1:67.

Gerrity, R. (1981) The role of the monocyte in atherogenesis: I. Transition of blood-borne monocytes into foam cells in fatty lesions. American Journal of Pathology 103(2):181-190.

Gersh, I. and H. Catchpole (1949) The organization of ground substance and basement membrane and its significance in tissue injury, disease and growth. American Journal of Anatomy 85:457-521.

Gey, K., H. Stahelin, and M. Eichholzer (1993) Poor plasma status of carotene and vitamin C is associated with higher mortality from ischemic heart disease and stroke: Basel Prospective Study. The Clinical Investigator 71(1):3-6.

Gillum, R., D. Ingram, and D. Makuc (1993) White blood cell count, coronary heart disease, and death: the NHANES I Epidemiologic Follow-up Study. American Heart Journal 125(3):855-863.

Ginter, E. (1970) Effect of dietary cholesterol on vitamin C metabolism in laboratory animals. Acta Medica Academiae Scientiarum Hungaricae 27(1):23-29.

Ginter, E., T. Kajaba, and O. Nizner (1970) The effect of ascorbic acid on cholesterolemia in healthy subjects with seasonal deficit of vitamin C. Nutrition and Metabolism 2(2):76-86.

Ginter, E., J. Cerven, R. Nemec, and L. Mikus (1971) Lowered cholesterol catabolism in guinea pigs with chronic ascorbic acid deficiency. American Journal of Clinical Nutrition 24(10):1238-1245.

Ginter, E. (1973) Cholesterol: vitamin C controls its transformation to bile acids. Science 179(74):702-704.

Ginter, E. (1975) The Role of Vitamin C in Cholesterol Catabolism and Atherogenesis. Bratislava, Czechoslovakia: Veda, Vydavatelstvo Slovenskej Akademie Vied.

Ginter, E. (1975a) Ascorbic acid in cholesterol and bile acid metabolism. Annals of the New York Academy of Sciences 258:410-421.

Ginter, E., O. Cerna, J. Budlovsky, V. Balaz, F. Hruba, V. Roch, and E. Sasko (1977) Effect of ascorbic acid on plasma cholesterol in humans in a long-term experiment. International Journal for Vitamin and Nutrition Research 47(2):123-134.

Ginter, E. (1978) Marginal vitamin C deficiency, lipid metabolism, and atherogenesis. Advances in Lipid Research 16:167-220.

Ginter, E., B. Zdichynec, O. Holzerova, E. Ticha, R. Kobza, M. Koziakova, O. Cerna, L. Ozdin, F. Hruba, V. Novakova, E. Sasko, and M. Gaher (1978) Hypocholesterolemic effect of ascorbic acid in maturity-onset diabetes mellitus. International Journal for Vitamin and Nutrition Research 48(4):368-373.

Golomb, B. (1998) Cholesterol and violence: is there a connection? Annals of Internal Medicine 128(6):478-487.

Golomb, B., H. Stattin, and S. Mednick (2000) Low cholesterol and violent crime. Journal of Psychiatric Research 34(4-5):301-309.

Gore, I., Y. Tanaka, T. Fujinami, and T. Shirahama (1965) Endothelial changes produced by ascorbic acid deficiency in guinea pigs. Archives of Pathology 80(4): 371-376.

Gould, B. (1958) Biosynthesis of collagen. III. The direct action of ascorbic acid on hydroxyproline and collagen formation in subcutaneous polyvinyl sponge implants in guinea pigs. The Journal of Biological Chemistry 232(2):637-649.

Gould, B. (1963) Collagen formation and fibrogenesis with special reference to the role of ascorbic acid. International Review of Cytology 15:301-354.

Green, S., J. Vowels, B. Waterman, S. Rothrock, and G. Kuniyoshi (1996) Leukocytosis: a new look at an old marker for acute myocardial infarction. Academic Emergency Medicine: Official Journal of the Society for Academic Emergency Medicine 3(11):1034-1041.

Greene, Jr., R., B. Houston, and S. Holleran (1995) Aggressiveness, dominance, developmental factors, and serum cholesterol level in college males. Journal of Behavioral Medicine 18(6):569-580.

Grossman, M., D. Dobrev, H. Himmel, U. Ravens, and W. Kirch (2001) Ascorbic acid-induced modulation of venous tone in humans. Hypertension 37(3):949-954.

Gudbjarnason, S., J. Fenton, P. Wolf, and R. Bing (1966) Stimulation of reparative processes following experimental myocardial infarction. Archives of Internal Medicine 118(1):33-40.

Gupta, M. and S. Chari (2005) Lipid peroxidation and antioxidant status in patients with diabetic retinopathy. Indian Journal of Physiology and Pharmacology 49(2): 187-192.

Gupta, M., P. Sharma, G. Garg, K. Kaur, G. Bedi, and A. Vij (2005) Plasma homocysteine: an independent or an interactive risk factor for coronary artery disease. Clinica Chimica Acta: International Journal of Clinical Chemistry 352(1-2):121-125.

Ha, T., M. Otsuka, and N. Arakawa (1990) The effect of graded doses of ascorbic acid on the tissue carnitine and plasma lipid concentrations. Journal of Nutritional Science and Vitaminology 36(3):227-234.

Haffner, S. (2005) Rationale for new American Diabetes Association Guidelines: are national cholesterol education program goals adequate for the patient with diabetes mellitus? The American Journal of Cardiology 96(4A):33E-36E.

Haim, M., V. Boyko, U. Goldbourt, A. Battler, and S. Behar (2004) Predictive value of elevated white blood cell count in patients with preexisting coronary heart disease: the Bezafibrate Infarction Prevention Study. Archives of Internal Medicine 164(4):433-439.

Hajishengallis, G., A. Sharma, M. Russell, and R. Genco (2002) Interactions of oral pathogens with toll-like receptors: possible role in atherosclerosis. Annals of Periodontology 7(1):72-78.

Hajjar, K. (2001) Homocysteine: a sulph'rous fire. The Journal of Clinical Investigation 107(6):663-664.

Hall, S. and G. Greendale (1998) The relation of dietary vitamin C intake to bone mineral density: results from the PEPI study. Calcified Tissue International 63(3):183-189.

Hamilton, I., W. Gilmore, I. Benzie, C. Mulholland, and J. Strain (2000) Interactions between vitamins C and E in human subjects. The British Journal of Nutrition 84(3): 261-267.

Harman, D. (1961) Atherosclerosis. Inhibiting effect of an antihistaminic drug, chlorpheniramine. Circulation Research 11:277-282.

Harman, D. (1963) Role of serum copper in coronary atherosclerosis. Circulation 28 (Abstract):658.

Hatanaka, H. and F. Egami (1976) Sulfate incorporation from ascorbate 2-sulfate into chondroitin sulfate by embryonic chick cartilage epiphyses. Journal of Biochemistry 80(6):1215-1221.

Haumer, M., J. Amighi, M. Exner, W. Mlekusch, S. Sabeti, O. Schlager, I. Schwarzinger, O. Wagner, E. Minar, and M. Schillinger (2005) Association of neutrophils and future cardiovascular events in patients with peripheral artery disease. Journal of Vascular Surgery: Official Publication, the Society for Vascular Surgery [and] International Society for Cardiovascular Surgery, North American Chapter 41(4):610-617.

Hayashi, E., J. Yamada, M. Kunitomo, M. Terada, T. Tomita, and T. Kinoshita (1976) Fundamental studies on physiological and pharmacological actions of L-ascorbate 2-sulfate. I. On the hypolipidemic effects. Journal of Nutritional Science and Vitaminology 22(3): 201-208.

Hayashi, E., J. Yamada, M. Kunitomo, M. Terada, and Y. Watanabe (1978) Fundamental studies on physiological and pharmacological actions of L-ascorbate 2-sulfate. VI. Effects of L-ascorbate 2-sulfate on lipid metabolism in guinea pigs. Japanese Journal of Pharmacology 28(1):133-143.

Heinecke, J., H. Rosen, and A. Chait (1984) Iron and copper promote modification of low density lipoprotein by human arterial smooth muscle cells in culture. The Journal of Clinical Investigation 74(5):1890-1894.

Hjerkinn, E., I. Seljeflot, L. Sandvik, I. Hjermann, and H. Arnesen (2005) Markers of endothelial cell activation in elderly men at high risk for coronary heart disease. Scandinavian Journal of Clinical and Laboratory Investigation 65(3):201-209.

Hofmann, M., E. Lalla, Y. Lu, M. Gleason, B. Wolf, N. Tanji, L. Ferran, Jr., B. Kohl, V. Rao, W. Kisiel, D. Stern, and A. Schmidt (2001) Hyperhomocysteinemia enhances vascular inflammation and accelerates atherosclerosis in a murine model. The Journal of Clinical Investigation 107(6):675-683.

Hollander, W., D. Kramsch, C. Franzblau, J. Paddock, and M. Colombo (1974) Suppression of atheromatous fibrous plaque formation by antiproliferative and anti-inflammatory drugs. Circulation Research 34 & 35(Suppl I):131-141.

Hopkins, P., L. Wu, S. Hunt, and E. Brinton (2005) Plasma triglycerides and type III hyperlipidemia are independently associated with premature familial coronary artery disease. Journal of the American College of Cardiology 45(7):1003-1012.

Horlick, L. and L. Katz (1949) Retrogression of atherosclerotic lesions on cessation of cholesterol feeding in the chick. Journal of Laboratory and Clinical Medicine 34:1427-1442.

Hovingh, G., B. Hutten, A. Holleboom, W. Petersen, P. Rol, A. Stalenhoef, A. Zwinderman, E. de Groot, J. Kastelein, and J. Kuivenhoven (2005) Compromised LCAT function is associated with increased atherosclerosis. Circulation 112(6):879-884.

Hu, W., P. Polinsky, E. Sadoun, M. Rosenfeld, and S. Schwartz (2005) Atherosclerotic lesions in the common coronary arteries of ApoE knockout mice. Cardiovascular Pathology: the Official Journal of the Society for Cardiovascular Pathology 14(3):120-125.

Huggins, H. (1993) It's All In Your Head. The Link Between Mercury Amalgams and Illness. Garden City Park, NY: Avery Publishing Group, Inc.

Huggins, H. and T. Levy (1999) Uninformed Consent: The Hidden Dangers in Dental Care. Charlottesville, VA: Hampton Roads Publishing Company, Inc.

Hume, R., E. Weyers, T. Rowan, D. Reid, and W. Hillis (1972) Leucocyte ascorbic acid levels after acute myocardial infarction. British Heart Journal 34(3):238-243.

Hume, R. and E. Weyers (1973) Changes in leucocyte ascorbic acid during the common cold. Scottish Medical Journal 18(1):3-7.

Hume, R., B. Vallance, and M. Muir (1982) Ascorbate status and fibrinogen concentrations after cerebrovascular accident. Journal of Clinical Pathology 35(2):195-199.

Humoller, F., M. Mockler, J. Holtnaus, and D. Mahler (1995) Enzymatic properties of ceruloplasmin. The Journal of Laboratory and Clinical Medicine 56:222-234.

Hunt, J., M. Bottoms, and M. Mitchinson (1992) Ascorbic acid oxidation: a potential cause of the elevated severity of atherosclerosis in diabetes mellitus? FEBS Letters 311(2):161-164.

Ilhan, F., H. Akbulut, I. Karaca, A. Godekmerdan, E. Ilkay, and V. Bulut (2005) Procalcitonin, C-reactive protein, and neopterin levels in patients with coronary atherosclerosis. Acta Cardiologica 60(4):361-365.

Inoue, K., Y. Kobayashi, H. Hanamura, and S. Toyokawa (2005) Association of periodontitis with increased white blood cell count and blood pressure. Blood Pressure 14(1):53-58.

Isles, C., D. Hole, C. Gillis, V. Hawthorne, and A. Lever (1989) Plasma cholesterol, coronary heart disease, and cancer in the Renfrew and Paisley survey. BMJ (Clinical Research Ed.) 298(6678):920-924.

Iso, H., T. Shimamoto, S. Sato, K. Koike, M. Iida, and Y. Komachi (1996) Passive smoking and plasma fibrinogen concentrations. American Journal of Epidemiology 144(12):1151-1154.

Issels, J. (1999) Cancer: A Second Opinion. Garden City Park, NY: Avery Publishing Group.

Izuka, K., K. Murata, K. Nakazawa, K. Okubo, and Y. Oshima (1968) Effects of chondroitin sulfates on serum lipids and hexosamines in atherosclerotic patients: with special reference to thrombus formation time. Japanese Heart Journal 9(5):453-460.

James, A., M. Knuiman, M. Divitini, A. Musk, and G. Ryan (1999) Associations between white blood cell count, lung function, respiratory illness and mortality: the Busselton Health Study. The European Respiratory Journal 13(5):1115-1119.

Janoff, A. (1985) Elastases and emphysema. Current assessment of the protease-antiprotease hypothesis. The American Review of Respiratory Disease 132(2): 417-433.

Jenkins, C. (1982) Psychosocial risk factors for coronary heart disease. Acta Medica Scandinavica. Supplementum 660:123-136.

Jialal, I., G. Vega, and S. Grundy (1990) Physiologic levels of ascorbate inhibit the oxidative modification of low density lipoprotein. Atherosclerosis 82(3):185-191.

Johnston, C., L. Martin, and X. Cai (1992) Antihistamine effect of supplemental ascorbic acid and neutrophil chemotaxis. Journal of the American College of Nutrition 11(2):172-176.

Johnston, C., R. Solomon, and C. Corte (1996) Vitamin C depletion is associated with alterations in blood histamine and plasma free carnitine in adults. Journal of the American College of Nutrition 15(6):586-591.

Jonas, B. and M. Mussolino (2000) Symptoms of depression as a prospective risk factor for stroke. Psychosomatic Medicine 62(4):463-471.

Jorde, L. and R. Williams (1988) Relation between family history of coronary artery disease and coronary risk variables. The American Journal of Cardiology 62(10 Pt 1):708-713.

Joshipura, K., F. Hu, J. Manson, M. Stampfer, E. Rimm, F. Speizer, G. Colditz, A. Ascherio, B. Rosner, D. Spiegelman, and W. Willett (2001) The effect of fruit and vegetable intake on risk for coronary heart disease. Annals of Internal Medicine 134(12):1106-1114.

Kagan, A., D. McGee, K. Yano, G. Rhoads, and A. Nomura (1981) Serum cholesterol and mortality in a Japanese-American population: the Honolulu Heart program. American Journal of Epidemiology 114(1):11-20.

Kalinina, A., L. Chazova, N. Perova, L. Pavlova, and V. Shchepkin (1993) [An increased risk of death from ischemic heart disease in men with low blood concentrations of total cholesterol and low-density lipoprotein cholesterol]. Russian. Terapevticheskii Arkhiv 65(4):27-32.

Kanani, P., C. Sinkey, R. Browning, M. Allaman, H. Knapp, and W. Haynes (1999) Role of oxidant stress in endothelial dysfunction produced by experimental hyperhomocyst(e)inemia in humans. Circulation 100(11):1161-1168.

Kannel, W., P. Wolf, W. Castelli, and R. D'Agostino (1987) Fibrinogen and risk of cardiovascular disease. The Framingham Study. The Journal of the American Medical Association 258(9):1183-1186.

Kapeghian, J. and A. Verlangieri (1984) The effects of glucose on ascorbic acid uptake in heart endothelial cells: possible pathogenesis of diabetic angiopathies. Life Sciences 34(6):577-584.

Karatzis, E., J. Lekakis, C. Papamichael, I. Andreadou, A. Cimponeriu, K. Aznaouridis, T. Papaioannou, A. Protogerou, and M. Mavrikakis (2005) Rapid effect of pravastatin on endothelial function and lipid peroxidation in unstable angina. International Journal of Cardiology 101(1):65-70.

Karjalainen, S., E. Soderling, L. Sewon, H. Lapinleimu, and O. Simell (2001) A prospective study on sucrose consumption, visible plaque and caries in children from 3 to 6 years of age. Community Dentistry and Oral Epidemiology 29(2):136-142.

Kark, J., A. Smith, and C. Hames (1980) The relationship of serum cholesterol to the incidence of cancer in Evans County, Georgia. Journal of Chronic Disease 33(5):311-332.

Karpen, C., S. Cataland, T. O'Dorisio, and R. Panganamala (1984) Interrelation of platelet vitamin E and thromboxane synthesis in type I diabetes mellitus. Diabetes 33(3):239-243.

Katz, E. (1996) Reduction of cholesterol and Lp(a) and regression of coronary artery disease: a case study. Journal of Orthomolecular Medicine 11(3):173-179.

Kaufmann, P., T. Gnecchi-Ruscone, M. di Terlizzi, K. Schafers, T. Luscher, and P. Camici (2000) Coronary heart disease in smokers: vitamin C restores coronary microcirculatory function. Circulation 102(11):1233-1238.

Kefalides, N. (1968) Isolation and characterization of the collagen from glomerular basement membrane. Biochemistry 7(9):3103-3112.

Kempler, P. (2005) Learning from large cardiovascular clinical trials: classical cardiovascular risk factors. Diabetes Research and Clinical Practice 68(Suppl 1): S43-47.

Keys, A., C. Aravanis, H. Blackburn, R. Buzina, A. Dontas, F. Fidanza, M. Karvonen, A. Menotti, S. Nedeljkovic, S. Punsar, et al. (1985) Serum cholesterol and cancer mortality in the Seven Countries Study. American Journal of Epidemiology 121(6):870-883.

Khatami, M., W. Li, and J. Rockey (1986) Kinetics of ascorbate transport by cultured retinal capillary pericytes. Inhibition by glucose. Investigative Ophthalmology & Visual Science 27(11):1665-1671.

Khaw, K. and P. Woodhouse (1995) Interrelation of vitamin C, infection, haemostatic factors, and cardiovascular disease. BMJ (Clinical Research ed.) 310(6994):1559-1563.

Khaw, K., S. Bingham, A. Welch, R. Luben, N. Wareham, S. Oakes, and N. Day (2001) Relation between plasma ascorbic acid and mortality in men and women in EPIC-Norfolk prospective study: a prospective population study. Lancet 357(9257):657-663.

Kiechl, S., G. Egger, M. Mayr, C. Wiedermann, E. Bonora, F. Oberhollenzer, M. Muggeo, Q. Xu, G. Wick, W. Poewe, and J. Willeit (2001) Chronic infections and the risk of carotid atherosclerosis. Prospective results from a large population study. Circulation 103(8):1064-1070.

King, C. and M. Menten (1935) The influence of vitamin C level upon resistance to diphtheria toxin. I. Changes in body weight and duration of life. Journal of Nutrition 10(2):129-139.

Kirk, J. and M. Dyrbye (1957) Mucopolysaccharides of human arterial tissue. II. Analysis of total isolated mucopolysaccharide material. Journal of Gerontology 12:23.

Kirk, J. (1959) Anticoagulant activity of human arterial mucopolysaccharides. Nature 184(4683):369-370.

Klein, H., S. Pich, S. Lindert, K. Nebendahl, P. Niedmann, and H. Kreuzer (1989) Combined treatment with vitamins E and C in experimental myocardial infarction in pigs. American Heart Journal 118(4):667-673.

Kleindienst, R., G. Schett, A. Amberger, C. Seitz, D. Michaelis, B. Metzler, H. Dietrich, Q. Xu, and G. Wick (1995) Atherosclerosis as an autoimmune condition. Israel Journal of Medical Sciences 31(10):596-599.

Klotz, O. (1906) A discussion of the classification and experimental production of arteriosclerosis. British Medical Journal 2:1767.

Klotz, O. (1906a) The relation of experimental arterial disease in animals to arteriosclerosis in man. Journal of Experimental Medicine, N.Y. 8:504.

Knekt, P., A. Reunanen, A. Aromaa, M. Heliovaara, T. Hakulinen, and M. Hakama (1988) Serum cholesterol and risk of cancer in a cohort of 39,000 men and women. Journal of Clinical Epidemiology 41(6):519-530.

Knekt, P., A. Reunanen, R. Jarvinen, R. Seppanen, M. Heliovaara, and A. Aromaa (1994) Antioxidant vitamin intake and coronary mortality in a longitudinal population study. American Journal of Epidemiology 139(12):1180-1189.

Kodama, M., T. Kodama, M. Murakami, and M. Kodama (1993) Diabetes mellitus is controlled by vitamin C treatment. In Vivo 7(6A):535-542.

Kodama, M., T. Kodama, M. Murakami, and M. Kodama (1994) Autoimmune disease and allergy are controlled by vitamin C treatment. In Vivo 8(2):251-257.

Kofoed, J. and W. Robertson (1966) Ascorbic acid and the synthesis of chondroitin sulfate. Biochimica et Biophysica Acta 124(1):86-94.

Kok, F., C. van Duijn, A. Hofman, G. Van der Voet, F. De Wolff, C. Paays, and H. Valkenburg (1988) Serum copper and zinc and the risk of death from cancer and cardiovascular diseases. American Journal of Epidemiology 128(2):352-359.

Kolovou, G., K. Anagnostopoulou, S. Daskalopoulou, D. Mikhailidis, and D. Cokkinos (2005) Clinical relevance of postprandial lipaemia. Current Medicinal Chemistry 12(17):1931-1945.

Kotronias, D. and N. Kapranos (2005) Herpes simplex virus as a determinant risk factor for coronary artery atherosclerosis and myocardial infarction. In Vivo (Athen, Greece) 19(2):351-357.

Krumdieck, C. and C. Butterworth (1974) Ascorbate-cholesterol-lecithin interactions: factors of potential importance in the pathogenesis of atherosclerosis. American Journal of Clinical Nutrition 27(8):866-876.

Ku, C., C. Yang, W. Lee, H. Chiang, C. Liu, and S. Lin (1999) Absence of a seasonal variation in myocardial infarction onset in a region without temperature extremes. Cardiology 89(4):277-282.

Kubzansky, L., I. Kawachi, A. Spiro, S. Weiss, P. Vokonas, and D. Sparrow (1997) Is worrying bad for your heart? A prospective study of worry and coronary heart disease in the Normative Aging Study. Circulation 95(4):818-824.

Kubzansky, L., I. Kawachi, S. Weiss, and D. Sparrow (1998) Anxiety and coronary heart disease: a synthesis of epidemiological, psychological, and experimental evidence. Annals of Behavioral Medicine 20(2):47-58.

Kubzansky, L. and I. Kawachi (2000) Going to the heart of the matter: do negative emotions cause coronary heart disease? Journal of Psychosomatic Research 48(4-5): 317-320.

Kugiyama, K., T. Motoyama, O. Hirashima, M. Ohgushi, H. Soejima, K. Misumi, H. Kawano, Y. Miyao, M. Yoshimura, H. Ogawa, T. Matsumura, S. Sugiyama, and H. Yasue (1998) Vitamin C attenuates abnormal vasomotor reactivity in spasm coronary arteries in patients with coronary spastic angina. Journal of the American College of Cardiology 32(1):103-109.

Kulacz, R. and T. Levy (2002) The Roots of Disease. Connecting Dentistry and Medicine. Philadelphia, PA: Xlibris Corporation.

Kurpesa, M., E. Trzos, and M. Krzeminska-Pakula (2003) White blood cell count and the occurrence of silent ischemia after myocardial infarction. Annals of Noninvasive Electrocardiology: the Official Journal of the International Society for Holter and Noninvasive Electrocardiology, Inc. 8(1):3-7.

Kwon, T., K. Kim, J. Ye, W. Lee, M. Moon, C. Joo, H. Lee, and Y. Kim (2004) Detection of enterovirus, cytomegalovirus, and Chlamydia pneumoniae in atheromas. Journal of Microbiology (Seoul, Korea) 42(4):299-304.

Laguesse, E. (1921) La structure lamelleuse et le developpement du tissu conjonctif lache chez les mammiferes en general et chez l'homme en particulier. Arch de Biol 31:173-298.

Langlois, M., D. Duprez, J. Delanghe, M. de Buyzere, and D. Clement. (2001) Serum vitamin C concentration is low in peripheral arterial disease and is associated with inflammation and severity of atherosclerosis. Circulation 103(14):1863-1868.

Lanman, T. and T. Ingalls (1937) Vitamin C deficiency and wound healing: an experimental and clinical study. Annals of Surgery 105(4):616-625.

Laskowski, H., A. Minczykowski, and H. Wysocki (1995) Mortality and clinical course of patients with acute myocardial infarction treated with streptokinase and antioxidants: mannitol and ascorbic acid. International Journal of Cardiology 48(3):235-237.

Lehr, H. and K. Arfors (1994) Mechanisms of tissue damage by leukocytes. Current Opinion in Hematology 1(1):92-99.

Lehr, H., B. Frei, and K. Arfors (1994) Vitamin C prevents cigarette smoke-induced leukocyte aggregation and adhesion to endothelium in vivo. Proceedings of the National Academy of Sciences of the United States of America 91(16):7688-7692.

Leite, P., M. Liberman, F. Sandoli de Brito, and F. Laurindo (2004) Redox processes underlying the vascular repair reaction. World Journal of Surgery 28(3):331-336.

Lemos, P., P. de Feyter, P. Serruys, F. Saia, C. Arampatzis, C. Disco, N. Mercado, V. Mainar, C. Moris, A. van den Bos, and G. Berghoefer (2005) Fluvastatin reduces the 4-year cardiac risk in patients with multivessel disease. International Journal of Cardiology 98(3):479-486.

Lenton, K., H. Therriault, A. Cantin, T. Fulop, H. Payette, and J. Wagner (2000) Direct correlation of glutathione and ascorbate and their dependence on age and season in human lymphocytes. The American Journal of Clinical Nutrition 71(5):1194-1200.

Leren, P. (1970) The Oslo Diet Heart Study: eleven-year report. Circulation 42(5):935-942.

Leskov, V. and I. Zatevakhin (2005) The role of the immune system in the pathogenesis of atherosclerosis [article in Russian]. Angiologiia i Sosudistaia Khirurgiia 11(2): 9-14.

Leveille, S., A. LaCroix, T. Koepsell, S. Beresford, G. Van Belle, and D. Buchner (1997) Dietary vitamin C and bone mineral density in postmenopausal women in Washington State, USA. Journal of Epidemiology and Community Health 51(5):479-485.

Levene, C. and J. Poole (1962) The collagen content of normal and atherosclerotic human aortic intima. British Journal of Experimental Pathology 43:469-471.

Levy, T. and H. Huggins (1996) Routine dental extractions routinely produce cavitations. Journal of Advancement in Medicine 9(4):235-249.

Levy, T. (2002) Vitamin C, Infectious Diseases, and Toxins. Curing the Incurable. Henderson: LivOn Books.

Licastro, F., G. Candore, D. Lio, E. Porcellini, G. Colonna-Romano, C. Franceschi, and C. Caruso (2005) Innate immunity and inflammation in ageing: a key for understanding age-related diseases. Immunity & Ageing 2:8.

Lindsay, S. and I. Chaikoff (1966) Naturally occurring arteriosclerosis in nonhuman primates. Journal of Atherosclerosis Research 6:36-61.

Lipid Research Clinics Program (1984) The Lipid Research Clinics Coronary Primary Prevention Trial results. I. Reduction in incidence of coronary heart disease. Journal of the American Medical Association 251(3): 351-374.

Liu, S., W. Willett, M. Stampfer, F. Hu, M. Franz, L. Sampson, C. Hennekens, and J. Manson (2000) A prospective study of dietary glycemic load, carbohydrate intake, and risk of coronary heart disease in US women. The American Journal of Clinical Nutrition 71(6):1455-1461.

Loh, H., A. Odumosu, and C. Wilson (1974) Factors influencing the metabolic availability of ascorbic acid. I. The effect of sex. Clinical Pharmacology and Therapeutics 16(2):390-408.

Loria, C., M. Klag, L. Caulfield, and P. Whelton (2000) Vitamin C status and mortality in US adults. The American Journal of Clinical Nutrition 72(1):139-145.

Loscalzo, J. (1996) The oxidant stress of hyperhomocyst(e)inemia. The Journal of Clinical Investigation 98(1):5-7.

Losonczy, K., T. Harris, and R. Havlik (1996) Vitamin E and vitamin C supplement use and risk of all-cause and coronary heart disease mortality in older persons: the Established Populations for Epidemiologic Studies of the Elderly. The American Journal of Clinical Nutrition 64(2):190-196.

Lynch, S., J. Gaziano, and B. Frei (1996) Ascorbic acid and atherosclerotic cardiovascular disease. Sub-cellular Biochemistry 25:331-367.

Lynch, S., H. Seftel, J. Torrance, R. Charlton, and T. Bothwell (1967) Accelerated oxidative catabolism of ascorbic acid in siderotic Bantu. The American Journal of Clinical Nutrition 20(6):641-647.

McBeath, M. and L. Pauling (1993) A case history: lysine/ ascorbate-related amelioration of angina pectoris. Journal of Orthomolecular Medicine 8(2):77-78.

McCall, M., J. van den Berg, F. Kuypers, D. Tribble, R. Krauss, L. Knoff, and T. Forte (1994) Modification of LCAT activity and HDL structure. New links between cigarette smoke and coronary heart disease risk. Arteriosclerosis and Thrombosis: A Journal of Vascular Biology 14(2):248-253.

McCormick, W. (1945) L'Union Medicale du Canada 74: 1205.

McCormick, W. (1957) Coronary thrombosis: a new concept of mechanism and etiology. Clinical Medicine July, pp. 839-845.

McCully, K. (1971) Homocysteine metabolism in scurvy, growth and arteriosclerosis. Nature 231(5302):391-392.

McMasters, P. and R. Parsons (1939) Physiological conditions existing in connective tissue. II. The state of the fluid in the intradermal tissue. Journal of Experimental Medicine 69:265-282.

MacCallum, P. (2005) Markers of hemostasis and systemic inflammation in heart disease and atherosclerosis in smokers. Proceedings of the American Thoracic Society 2(1):34-43.

Machtey, I., I. Syrkis, and M. Fried (1975) Studies of blood ascorbic acid levels in acute myocardial infarction. Clinica Chimica Acta 62(1):149-151.

Maeda, N., H. Hagihara, Y. Nakata, S. Hiller, J. Wilder, and R. Reddick (2000) Aortic wall damage in mice unable to synthesize ascorbic acid. Proceedings of the National Academy of Sciences of the United States of America 97(2):841-846.

Mainous, A., B. Wells, R. Koopman, C. Everett, and J. Gill (2005) Iron, lipids, and risk of cancer in the Framingham Offspring cohort. American Journal of Epidemiology 161(12):1115-1122.

Majno, G. and G. Palade (1961) Studies on inflammation. I. The effect of histamine and serotonin on vascular permeability: an electron microscopic study. The Journal of Biophysical and Biochemical Cytology 11: 571-605.

Majno, G., G. Palade, and G. Schoefl (1961) Studies on inflammation. II. The site of action of histamine and serotonin along the vascular tree: a topographic study. The Journal of Biophysical and Biochemical Cytology 11:607-626.

Mak, S. and G. Newton (2001) Vitamin C augments the inotropic response to dobutamine in humans with normal left ventricular function. Circulation 103(6):826-830.

Makita, S., M. Nakamura, and K. Hiramori (2005) The association of C-reactive protein levels with carotid intima-media complex thickness and plaque formation in the general population. Stroke: a Journal of Cerebral Circulation 36(10):2138-2142.

Malhotra, S., G. Tesar, and K. Franco (2000) The relationship between depression and cardiovascular disorders. Current Psychiatry Reports 2(3):241-246.

Mann, G., S. Andrus, A. McNally, and F. Stare (1953) Journal of Experimental Medicine 98:195.

Mann, G. (1974) Hypothesis: the role of vitamin C in diabetic angiopathy. Perspectives in Biology and Medicine 17(2):210-217.

Mann, G. and P. Newton (1975) The membrane transport of ascorbic acid. Annals of the New York Academy of Sciences 258:243-252.

Manthey, J., M. Stoeppler, W. Morgenstern, E. Nussel, D. Opherk, A. Weintraut, and W. Kubler (1981) Magnesium and trace metals: risk factors for coronary heart disease? Association between blood levels and angiographic findings. Circulation 64(4):722-729.

Manttari, M., V. Manninen, P. Koskinen, J. Huttunen, E. Oksanen, L. Tenkanen, O. Heinonen, and M. Frick (1992) Leukocytes as a coronary risk factor in a dyslipidemic male population. American Heart Journal 123(4 Pt 1):873-877.

Marcinko, D., M. Martinac, D. Karlovic, I. Filipcic, C. Loncar, N. Pivac, and M. Jakovljevic (2005) Are there differences in serum cholesterol and cortisol concentrations between violent and non-violent schizophrenic male suicide attempters? Collegium Antropologicum 29(1):153-157.

Maritz, G. (1996) Ascorbic acid. Protection of lung tissue against damage. Subcellular Biochemistry 25:265-291.

Marone, G., M. Gentile, A. Petraroli, N. de Rosa, and M. Triggiani (2001) Histamine-induced activation of human lung macrophages. International Archives of Allergy and Immunology 124(1-3):249-252.

Mastellone, I., E. Polichetti, S. Gres, C. de la Maisonneuve, N. Domingo, V. Marin, Anne-Marie Lorec, C. Farnarier, H. Portugal, G. Kaplanski, and F. Chanussot (2000) Dietary soybean phosphatidylcholines lower lipidemia: Mechanisms at the levels of intestine, endothelial cell, and hepato-biliary axis. Journal of Nutritional Biochemistry 11(9):461-466.

Matsushima, T., Y. Nakashima, M. Sugano, H. Tasaki, A. Kuroiwa, and O. Koide (1987) Suppression of atherogenesis in hypercholesterolemic rabbits by chondroitin-6-sulfate. Artery 14(6):316-337.

Maxwell, S. (2000) Coronary artery disease—free radical damage, antioxidant protection and the role of homocysteine. Basic Research in Cardiology 95(Suppl 1):I65-I71.

May, J. (2000) How does ascorbic acid prevent endothelial dysfunction? Free Radical Biology & Medicine 28(9): 1421-1429.

May, J. and Z. Qu (2005) Transport and intracellular accumulation of vitamin C in endothelial cells: relevance to collagen synthesis. Archives of Biochemistry and Biophysics 434(1):178-186.

Mayr, M., B. Metzler, S. Kiechl, J. Willeit, G. Schett, Q. Xu, and G. Wick (1999) Endothelial cytotoxicity mediated by serum antibodies to heat shock proteins of Escherichia coli and Chlamydia pneumoniae: immune reactions to heat shock proteins as a possible link between infection and atherosclerosis. Circulation 99(12):1560-1566.

Mazur, A., S. Green, and A. Carleton (1960) Mechanism of plasma iron incorporation into hepatic ferritin. Journal of Biological Chemistry 235:595.

Meier, C., S. Jick, L. Derby, C. Vasilakis, and H. Jick (1998) Acute respiratory-tract infections and risk of first-time acute myocardial infarction. Lancet 351(9114):1467-1471.

Meinig, G. (1996) Root Canal Cover-Up. Ojai, CA: Bion Publishing.

Melhus, H., K. Michaelsson, L. Holmberg, A. Wolk, and S. Ljunghall (1999) Smoking, antioxidant vitamins, and the risk of hip fracture. Journal of Bone and Mineral Research 14(1):129-135.

Melnick, J., E. Adam, and M. DeBakey (1995) Cytomegalovirus and atherosclerosis. Bioessays 17(10): 899-903.

Mennander, A., T. Angervuori, H. Huhtala, P. Karhunen, M. Tarkka, and P. Kuukasjarvi (2005) Positive family history of coronary atherosclerosis and serum triglycerides may predict repeated coronary artery bypass surgery. Scandinavian Cardiovascular Journal: SCJ 39(4):225-228.

Mennoti, A., D. Kromhout, H. Blackburn, D. Jacobs, and M. Lanti (2004) Forty-year mortality from cardiovascular diseases and all causes of death in the US Railroad cohort of the Seven Countries Study. European Journal of Epidemiology 19(5):417-424.

Menten, M. and C. King (1935) The influence of vitamin C level upon resistance to diphtheria toxin. II. Production of diffuse hyperplastic arteriosclerosis and degeneration in various organs. Journal of Nutrition 10(2):141-153.

Mickle, D., R. Li, R. Weisel, P. Birnbaum, T. Wu, G. Jackowski, M. Madonik, G. Burton, and K. Ingold (1989) Myocardial salvage with trolox and ascorbic acid for an acute evolving infarction. The Annals of Thoracic Surgery 47(4):553-557.

Minick, C., C. Fabricant, J. Fabricant, and M. Litrenta (1979) Atheroarteriosclerosis induced by infection with a herpesvirus. American Journal of Pathology 96(3): 673-706.

Minqin, R., F. Watt, B. Huat, and B. Halliwell (2003) Correlation of iron and zinc levels with lesion depth in newly formed atherosclerotic lesions. Free Radical Biology & Medicine 34(6):746-752.

Moon, H. and J. Rinehart (1952) Histogenesis of coronary arteriosclerosis. Circulation 6(4):481-488.

Mooradian, A. and J. Morley (1987) Micronutrient status in diabetes mellitus. The American Journal of Clinical Nutrition 45(5):877-895.

Moran, J., L. Cohen, J. Greene, G. Xu, E. Feldman, C. Hames, and D. Feldman (1993) Plasma ascorbic acid concentrations relate inversely to blood pressure in human subjects. The American Journal of Clinical Nutrition 57(2):213-217.

Morgan, A., H. Gillum, and R. Williams (1955) Nutritional status of the aging. III. Serum ascorbic acid and intake. Journal of Nutrition 55:431-448.

Morita, H., Y. Saito, N. Ohashi, M. Yoshikawa, M. Katoh, T. Ashida, H. Kurihara, T. Nakamura, M. Kurabayashi, and R. Nagai (2005) Fluvastatin ameliorates the hyperhomocysteinemia-induced endothelial dysfunction: the antioxidative properties of fluvastatin. Circulation Journal: Offician Journal of the Japanese Circulation Society 69(4):475-480.

Morris, K. and M. Zemel (1999) Glycemic index, cardiovascular disease, and obesity. Nutrition Reviews 57(9 Pt 1):273-276.

Morrison, L., O. Schjeide, J. Quilligan, et al. (1963) Effects of acid mucopolysaccharides on growth rates and constituent lipids of tissue cultures. Proceedings of the Society for Experimental Biology and Medicine 113: 362-366.

Morrison, L., O. Schjeide, J. Quilligan, et al. (1965) Metabolic parameters in the growth-stimulating effect of chondroitin sulfate A in tissue cultures. Proceedings of the Society for Experimental Biology and Medicine 119:618-622.

Morrison, L., K. Murata, J. Quilligan, O. Schjeide, and L. Freeman (1966) Prevention of atherosclerosis in sub-human primates by chondroitin sulfate A. Circulation Research 19(2):358-363.

Morrison, L. (1968) Treatment of coronary arteriosclerotic heart disease with chondroitin sulfate-A: preliminary report. Journal of the American Geriatrics Society 16(7): 779-785.

Morrison, L. (1971) Reduction of ischemic coronary heart disease by chondroitin sulfate A. Angiology 22(3):165-174.

Morrison, L., G. Bajwa, R. Alfin-Slater, and B. Ershoff (1972) Prevention of vascular lesions by chondroitin sulfate A in the coronary artery and aorta of rats induced by a hypervitaminosis D, cholesterol-containing diet. Atherosclerosis 16(1):105-118.

Morrow, D. and P. Ridker (2000) C-reactive protein, inflammation, and coronary risk. Medical Clinics of North America 84(1):149-161, ix.

Morton, D., E. Barrett-Connor, and D. Schneider (2001) Vitamin C supplement use and bone mineral density in postmenopausal women. Journal of Bone and Mineral Research 16(1):135-140.

Muhlestein, J. (2000) Infectious agents, antibiotics, and coronary artery disease. Current Interventional Cardiology Reports 2(4):342-348.

Murata, K. (1962) Inhibitory effects of chondroitin polysulphate on lipemia and atherosclerosis in connection with its anticoagulant activity. Naturewissenschaften 49:39-40.

Myasnikov, A. (1958) Influence of some factors on development of experimental cholesterol atherosclerosis. Circulation 17:99-113.

Nakazawa, K., K. Murata, K. Izuka, and Y. Oshima (1969) The short-term effects of chondroitin sulfates A and C on coronary atherosclerotic subjects: with reference to its anti-thrombogenic activities. Japanese Heart Journal 10(4):289-296.

Nakazawa, K. and K. Murata (1975) Long term effects of chondroitin sulphates A and C on atherosclerotic subjects. Zeitschrift fur Alternsforschung 29(4):385-389.

Nakazawa, K. and K. Murata (1978) The therapeutic effect of chondroitin polysulphate in elderly atherosclerotic patients. Journal of International Medical Research 6(3):217-225.

Nappo, F., N. de Rosa, R. Marfella, D. de Lucia, D. Ingrosso, A. Perna, B. Farzati, and D. Giugliano (1999) Impairment of endothelial functions by acute hyperhomocysteinemia and reversal by antioxidant vitamins. Journal of the American Medical Association 281(22):2113-2118.

Ness, A., D. Chee, and P. Elliott (1997) Vitamin C and blood pressure—an overview. Journal of Human Hypertension 11(6):343-350.

Ness, A., K. Khaw, S. Bingham, and N. Day (1996a) Vitamin C status and serum lipids. European Journal of Clinical Nutrition 50(11):724-729.

Ness, A., K. Khaw, S. Bingham, and N. Day (1996) Vitamin C status and blood pressure. Journal of Hypertension 14(4):503-508.

Newman, H. and D. Zilversmit (1962) Quantitative aspects of cholesterol flux in rabbit atheromatous lesions. Journal of Biological Chemistry 237(7):2078-2084.

Newton, H., C. Schorah, N. Habibzadeh, D. Morgan, and R. Hullin (1985) The cause and correction of low blood vitamin C concentrations in the elderly. The American Journal of Clinical Nutrition 42(4):656-659.

Nicholson, A. and D. Hajjar (1999) Herpesviruses and thrombosis: activation of coagulation on the endothelium. Clinica Chimica Acta (International Journal of Clinical Chemistry) 286(1-2):23-29.

Niendorf, A., M. Rath, K. Wolk, et al. (1990) Morphological detection and quantification of lipoprotein(a) deposition in atheromatous lesions of human aorta and coronary arteries. Virchows Arch A, Pathological Anatomy and Histopathology 417(2):105-111.

Norum, K., S. Borsting, and I. Grundt (1970) Familial lecithin:cholesterol acyltransferase deficiency. Study of two new patients and their close relatives. Acta Medica Scandinavica 188(4):323-326.

Nygard, O., J. Nordrehaug, H. Refsum, P. Ueland, M. Farstad, and S. Vollset (1997) Plasma homocysteine levels and mortality in patients with coronary artery disease. The New England Journal of Medicine 337(4): 230-236.

Nyyssonen, K., M. Parviainen, R. Salonen, J. Tuomilehto, and J. Salonen (1997) Vitamin C deficiency and risk of myocardial infarction: prospective population study of men from eastern Finland. BMJ 314(7081):634-638.

O'Connor, C., P. Gurbel, and V. Serebruany (2000) Depression and ischemic heart disease. American Heart Journal 140(4 Suppl):63-69.

Ogawa, K., K. Ueda, H. Sasaki, H. Yamasaki, K. Okamoto, H. Wakasaki, E. Matsumoto, H. Furuta, T. Hanabusa, M. Nishi, and K. Nanjo (2004) History of obesity as a risk factor for both carotid atherosclerosis and microangiopathy. Diabetes Research and Clinical Practice 66(Suppl 1):S165-S168.

Ohlwiler, D., M. Jurkiewicz, H. Butcher, and J. Brown (1960) The effect of heparin and ascorbic acid upon the formation of collagen. Surgical Forum 10:301-303.

Omland, T., A. Samuelsson, M. Hartford, J. Herlitz, T. Karlsson, B. Christensen, and K. Caidahl (2000) Serum homocysteine concentration as an indicator of survival in patients with acute coronary syndromes. Archives of Internal Medicine 160(12):1834-1840.

Orio, F., S. Palomba, T. Cascella, S. Di Biase, F. Manguso, L. Tauchmanova, L. Nardo, D. Labella, S. Savastano, T. Russo, F. Zullo, A. Colao, and G. Lombardi (2005) The increase of leukocytes as a new putative marker of low-grade chronic inflammation and early cardiovascular risk in polycystic ovary syndrome. The Journal of Clinical Endocrinology and Metabolism 90(1):2-5.

Ornato, J., M. Peberdy, N. Chandra, and D. Bush (1996) Seasonal pattern of acute myocardial infarction in the National Registry of Myocardial Infarction. Journal of the American College of Cardiology 28(7):1684-1688.

Osaki, S., J. McDermott, and E. Frieden (1964) Proof of the ascorbate oxidase activity of ceruloplasmin. The Journal of Biological Chemistry 239:3570-3575.

Owens, G. and T. Hollis (1979) Relationship between inhibition of aortic histamine formation, aortic albumin permeability and atherosclerosis. Atherosclerosis 34(4): 365-373.

Ozmen, D., B. Boydak, I. Mutaf, M. Zoghi, K. Kumanlioglu, I. Guner, and O. Bayindir (1999) The state of lipid peroxidation and antioxidants following thrombolytic therapy with rt-PA and streptokinase in acute myocardial infarction. Japanese Heart Journal 40(3):267-273.

Palatini, P. and S. Julius (2004) Elevated heart rate: a major risk factor for cardiovascular disease. Clinical and Experimental Hypertension 26(7-8):637-644.

Palinski, W., S. Yla-Herttuala, M. Rosenfeld, S. Butler, S. Socher, S. Parthasarathy, L. Curtiss, and J. Witztum (1990) Antisera and monoclonal antibodies specific for epitopes generated during oxidative modification of low density lipoprotein. Arteriosclerosis 10(3):325-335.

Paramo, J., O. Beloqui, C. Roncal, A. Benito, and J. Orbe (2004) Validation of plasma fibrinogen as a marker of carotid atherosclerosis in subjects free of clinical cardiovascular disease. Haematologica 89(10):1226-1231.

Parissis, J., K. Fountoulaki, I. Paraskevaidis, and D. Kremastinos (2005) Depression in chronic heart failure: novel pathophysiological mechanisms and therapeutic approaches. Expert Opinion on Investigational Drugs 14(5):567-577.

Park, K., H. Yang, H. Kim, Y. Lee, H. Hur, J.S. Kim, B. Koo, M. Han, J.H. Kim, Y. Jeong, and J.S. Kim (2005) Low density lipoprotein inactivates Vibrio vulnificus cytolysin through the oligomerization of toxin monomer. Medical Microbiology and Immunology 194(3):137-141.

Paterson, J. (1936) Vascularization and hemorrhage of the intima of arteriosclerotic coronary arteries. Archives of Pathology 22:313-324.

Paterson, J. (1938) Capillary rupture with intimal hemorrhage as a causative factor in coronary thrombosis. Archives of Pathology 25:474-487.

Paterson, J. (1941) Some factors in the causation of intimal hemorrhages and in the precipitation of coronary thrombi. Canadian Medical Association Journal 44:114-120.

Pauling, L. (1983) Vitamin C and longevity. Agressologie 24(7):317-319.

Pauling, L. (1991) Case report: lysine/ascorbate-related amelioration of angina pectoris. Journal of Orthomolecular Medicine 6(3&4):144-146.

Pauling, L. (1993) Third case report on lysine-ascorbate amelioration of angina pectoris. Journal of Orthomolecular Medicine 8(3):137-138.

Pauling, L. (1994) Linus Pauling: the last interview. British Journal of Optimum Nutrition August.

Pekkala, E., E. Hietala, M. Puukka, and M. Larmas (2000) Effects of a high sucrose diet and intragastric sucrose feeding on the dentinogenesis, dental caries, and mineral excretion of the young rat. Acta Odontologica Scandinavica 58(4):155-159.

Pelletier, O., (1975) Vitamin C and cigarette smokers. Annals of the New York Academy of Sciences 258:156-167.

Pelletier, O. (1977) Vitamin C and tobacco. International Journal for Vitamin and Nutrition Research. Supplement 16:147.

Piatti, P. and L. Monti (2005) Insulin resistance, hyperleptinemia and endothelial dysfunction in coronary restenosis. Current Opinion in Pharmacology 5(2):160-164.

Piedrola, G., E. Novo, F. Escobar, and R. Garcia-Robles (2001) White blood count and insulin resistance in patients with coronary artery disease. Annales d'Endocrinologie 62(1 Pt 1):7-10.

Pirani, C. and H. Catchpole (1951) Serum glycoproteins in experimental scurvy. A.M.A. Archives of Pathology 51: 597-601.

Pirani, C. and S. Levenson (1953) Effect of vitamin C deficiency on healed wounds. Proceedings of the Society for Experimental Biology and Medicine 82:95-99.

Pleiner, J., F. Mittermayer, G. Schaller, C. Marsik, R. MacAllister, and M. Wolzt (2003) Inflammation-induced vasoconstrictor hyporeactivity is caused by oxidative stress. Journal of the American College of Cardiology 42(9):1656-1662.

Poal-Manresa, J., K. Little, and J. Trueta (1970) Some observations on the effects of vitamin C deficiency on bone. British Journal of Experimental Pathology 51(4): 372-378.

Polichetti, E., N. Diaconescu, P. de la Porte, L. Malli, H. Portugal, A. Pauli, H. Lafont, B. Tuchweber, I. Yousef, and F. Chanussot (1996) Cholesterol-lowering effect of soyabean lecithin in normolipidaemic rats by stimulation of biliary lipid secretion. British Journal of Nutrition 75(3):471-478.

Polichetti, E., A. Janisson, P. de la Porte, H. Portugal, J. Leonardi, A. Luna, P. La Droitte, and F. Chanussot (2000) Dietary polyenylphosphatidylcholine decreases cholesterolemia in hypercholesterolemic rabbits: role of the hepato-biliary axis. Life Sciences 67(21):2563-2576.

Preston, A., C. Rodriguez, C. Rivera, and H. Sahai (2003) Influence of environmental tobacco smoke on vitamin C status in children. The American Journal of Clinical Nutrition 77(1):167-172.

Price, K., C. Price, and R. Reynolds (1996) Hyperglycemia-induced latent scurvy and atherosclerosis: the scorbutic-metaplasia hypothesis. Medical Hypotheses 46(2):119-129.

Priest, R. (1970) Formation of epithelial basement membrane is restricted by scurvy in vitro and is stimulated by vitamin C. Nature 225(234):744-745.

Punsar, S., O. Erametsa, M. Karvonen, A. Ryhanen, P. Hilska, and H. Vornamo (1975) Coronary heart disease and drinking water. A search in two Finnish male cohorts for epidemiologic evidence of a water factor. Journal of Chronic Diseases 28(5-6):259-287.

Qutob, S., S. Dixon, and J. Wilson (1998) Insulin stimulates vitamin C recycling and ascorbate accumulation in osteoblastic cells. Endocrinology 139(1):51-56.

Rajasekhar, D., P. Srinivasa Rao, S. Latheef, K. Saibaba, and G. Subramanyam (2004) Association of serum antioxidants and risk of coronary heart disease in South Indian population. Indian Journal of Medical Sciences 58(11):465-471.

Ramirez, J. and N. Flowers (1980) Leukocyte ascorbic acid and its relationship to coronary artery disease in man. The American Journal of Clinical Nutrition 33(10):2079-2087.

Rasouli, M., K. Nasir, R. Blumenthal, R. Park, D. Aziz, and M. Budoff (2005) Plasma homocysteine predicts progression of atherosclerosis. Atherosclerosis 181(1):159-165.

Rath, M., A. Niendorf, T. Reblin, M. Dietel, H. Krebber, and U. Beisiegel (1989) Detection and quantification of lipoprotein(a) in the arterial wall of 107 coronary bypass patients. Arteriosclerosis 9(5):579-592.

Rath, M. and L. Pauling (1990) Hypothesis: lipoprotein(a) is a surrogate for ascorbate. Proceedings of the National Academy of Science USA 87(16):6204-6207.

Rath, M. and L. Pauling (1990a) Immunological evidence for the accumulation of lipoprotein(a) in the atherosclerotic lesion of the hypoascorbemic guinea pig. Proceedings of the National Academy of Science USA 87(23):9388-9390.

Rath, M. and L. Pauling (1991) Solution to the puzzle of human cardiovascular disease: its primary cause is ascorbate deficiency leading to the deposition of lipoprotein(a) and fibrinogen/fibrin in the vascular wall. Journal of Orthomolecular Medicine 6(3&4):125-134.

Rath, M. and L. Pauling (1991a) Apoprotein(a) is an adhesive protein. Journal of Orthomolecular Medicine 6(3&4):139-143.

Rath, M. (1992) Reducing the risk for cardiovascular disease with nutritional supplements. Journal of Orthomolecular Medicine 7(3):153-162.

Rath, M. and A. Niedzwiecki (1996) Nutritional supplement program halts progression of early coronary atherosclerosis documented by ultrafast computed tomography. Journal of Applied Nutrition 48(3):68-78.

Rauch, U., J. Osende, V. Fuster, J. Badimon, Z. Fayad, and J. Chesebro (2001) Thrombus formation on atherosclerotic plaques: pathogenesis and clinical consequences. Annals of Internal Medicine 134(3):224-238.

Rehema, A., M. Zilmer, K. Zilmer, T. Kullisaar, and T. Vihalemm (1998) Could long-term alimentary iron overload have an impact on the parameters of oxidative stress? A study on the basis of a village in southern Estonia. Annals of Nutrition & Metabolism 42(1):40-43.

Reinehr, T. and W. Andler (2004) Changes in the atherogenic risk factor profile according to degree of weight loss. Archives of Diseases in Childhood 89(5): 419-422.

Ridker, P., N. Rifai, M. Pfeffer, F. Sacks, and E. Braunwald (1999) Long-term effects of pravastatin on plasma concentration of C-reactive protein. The Cholesterol and Recurrent Events (CARE) Investigators. Circulation 100(3):230-235.

Ridker, P., N. Rifai, and S. Lowenthal (2001) Rapid reduction in C-reactive protein with cerivastatin among 785 patients with primary hypercholesterolemia. Circulation 103(9):1191-1193.

Riemersma, R., D. Wood, C. Macintyre, R. Elton, K. Gey, and M. Oliver (1991) Risk of angina pectoris and plasma concentrations of vitamins A, C, and E and carotene. Lancet 337(8732):1-5.

Robicsek, F. and M. Thubrikar (1994) The freedom from atherosclerosis of intramyocardial coronary arteries: reduction of mural stress—a key factor. European Journal of Cardio-thoracic Surgery: Official Journal of the European Association for Cardio-thoracic Surgery 8(5):228-235.

Rodriguez, B. (2001) Both high and low cholesterol linked to increased CHD risk in elderly men. Presented at the American Heart Association's 41st Annual Conference on Cardiovascular Disease Epidemiology and Prevention, San Antonio, TX, March 6.

Roose, S. and E. Spatz (1999) Treatment of depression in patients with heart disease. The Journal of Clinical Psychiatry 60(Suppl 20):34-37.

Ross, R. (1992) The pathogenesis of atherosclerosis. In: Braunwald, E. (ed.) Heart Disease: A Textbook of Cardiovascular Medicine. Philadelphia, PA: W.B. Saunders Company.

Ross, R. (1993) Rous-Whipple Award Lecture. Atherosclerosis: a defense mechanism gone awry. American Journal of Pathology 143(4):987-1002.

Rowan, P., D. Haas, J. Campbell, D. Maclean, and K. Davidson (2005) Depressive symptoms have an independent, gradient risk for coronary heart disease incidence in a random, population-based sample. Annals of Epidemiology 15(4):316-320.

Rumsey, S., R. Daruwala, H. Al-Hasani, M. Zarnowski, I. Simpson, and M. Levine (2000) Dehydroascorbic acid transport by GLUT4 in Xenopus oocytes and isolated rat adipocytes. The Journal of Biological Chemistry 275(36):28246-28253.

Ruskin, S. (1938) Studies of the parallel action of vitamin C and calcium. American Journal of Digestive Diseases 5: 408-411.

Rutenberg, H. and L. Soloff (1971) Possible mechanism of egress of free cholesterol from the arterial wall. Nature 230(5289):123-125.

Sadava, D., D. Watumull, K. Sanders, and K. Downey (1982) The effect of vitamin C on the rapid induction of aortic changes in rabbits. Journal of Nutritional Science and Vitaminology 28(2):85-92.

Sagun, K., J. Carcamo, and D. Golde (2005) Vitamin C enters mitochondria via facilitative glucose transporter 1 (Glut1) and confers mitochondrial protection against oxidative injury. The FASEB Journal: Official Publication of the Federation of American Societies for Experimental Biology 19(12):1657-1667.

Sahyoun, N., P. Jacques, and R. Russell (1996) Carotenoids, vitamins C and E, and mortality in an elderly population. American Journal of Epidemiology 144(5): 501-511.

Sakai, N., T. Yokoyama, C. Date, N. Yoshiike, and Y. Matsumura (1998) An inverse relationship between serum vitamin C and blood pressure in a Japanese community. Journal of Nutritional Science and Vitaminology 44(6):853-867.

Salnikow, K. and K. Kasprzak (2005) Ascorbate depletion: a critical step in nickel carcinogenesis? Environmental Health Perspectives 113(5):577-584.

Salonen, J., G. Alfthan, J. Huttunen, J. Pikkarainen, and P. Puska (1982) Association between cardiovascular death and myocardial infarction and serum selenium in a matched-pair longitudinal study. Lancet 2(8291):175-179.

Salonen, J., R. Salonen, H. Korpela, S. Suntioinen, and J. Tuomilehto (1991) Serum copper and the risk of acute myocardial infarction: a prospective population study of men in eastern Finland. American Journal of Epidemiology 134(3):268-276.

Salonen, J., K. Nyyssonen, H. Korpela, J. Tuomilehto, R. Seppanen, and R. Salonen (1992) High stored iron levels are associated with excess risk of myocardial infarction in eastern Finnish men. Circulation 86(3):803-811.

Salter, W. and J. Aub (1931) Studies of calcium and phosphorus metabolism. IX. Deposition of calcium in bone in healing scorbutus. Archives of Pathology 11:380-382.

Sankaran, G. and B. Krishnan (1936) Observations on the heart rate in vitamin B1 and C deficiency. The Indian Journal of Medical Research 23(3):747-754.

Santamarina-Fojo, S., G. Lambert, J. Hoeg, and H. Brewer Jr. (2000) Lecithin-cholesterol acyltransferase: role in lipoprotein metabolism, reverse cholesterol transport and atherosclerosis. Current Opinion in Lipidology 11(3):267-275.

Sarji, K., J. Kleinfelder, P. Brewington, J. Gonzalez, H. Hempling, and J. Colwell (1979) Decreased platelet vitamin C in diabetes mellitus: possible role in hyperaggregation. Thrombosis Research 15(5/6):639-650.

Sato, Y., N. Hotta, N. Sakamoto, S. Matsuoka, N. Ohishi, and K. Yagi (1979) Lipid peroxide level in plasma of diabetic patients. Biochemical Medicine 21(1):104-107.

Scanu, A., D. Pfaffinger, J. Lee, and J. Hinman (1994) A single point mutation (Trp72Arg) in human apo(a) kringle 4-37 associated with a lysine binding defect in Lp(a). Biochimica et Biophysica Acta 1227(1-2):41-45.

Schatzkin, A., R. Hoover, R. Taylor, R. Ziegler, C. Carter, D. Larson, and L. Licitra (1987) Serum cholesterol and cancer in the NHANES I epidemiologic followup study. National Health and Nutrition Examination Study. Lancet 2(8554):298-301.

Scher, A. (2000) Absence of atherosclerosis in human intramyocardial coronary arteries: a neglected phenomenon. Atherosclerosis 149(1):1-3.

Schorah, C., A. Newill, D. Scott, and D. Morgan (1979) Clinical effects of vitamin C in elderly inpatients with low blood-vitamin-C levels. Lancet 1(8113):403-405.

Schwartz, E. and L. Adamy (1976) Effect of ascorbic acid on arylsulfatase A and B activities in human chondrocyte cultures. Connective Tissue Research 4(4):211-218.

Schwartz, E. and L. Adamy (1977) Effect of ascorbic acid on arylsulfatase activities and sulfated proteoglycan metabolism in chondrocytes cultures. The Journal of Clinical Investigation 60(1):96-106.

Seccareccia, F., F. Pannozzo, F. Dima, A. Minoprio, A. Menditto, C. Lo Noce, and S. Giampaoli (2001) Heart rate as a predictor of mortality: the MATISS project. American Journal of Public Health 91(8):1258-1263.

Seymour, J. and E. Sowton (1964) Action of ascorbic acid on digitalis effects in the cardiogram. British Medical Journal 1:1551-1552.

Shafar, J. (1967) Rapid reversion of electrocardiographic abnormalities after treatment in two cases of scurvy. Lancet 2(7508):176-178.

Shaffer, C. (1944) The diuretic effect of ascorbic acid. Preliminary report on its use in cardiac decompensation. The Journal of the American Medical Association 124(11):700-701.

Shaffer, C. (1970) Ascorbic acid and atherosclerosis. American Journal of Clinical Nutrition 23(1):27-30.

Shah, S. and M. Alam (2003) Role of iron in atherosclerosis. American Journal of Kidney Diseases: the Official Journal of the National Kidney Foundation 41(3 Suppl 1):S80-S83.

Shannon, I. (1973) Significant correlations between gingival scores and ascorbic acid status. Journal of Dental Research 52(2):394.

Sher, L. (2000) The possible effect of seasonal mood changes on the seasonal distribution of myocardial infarction. Medical Hypotheses 54(6):861-863.

Sherry, S. and E. Ralli (1948) Further studies of the effects of insulin on the metabolism of vitamin C. Journal of Clinical Investigation 27:217-225.

Sheth, T., C. Nair, J. Muller, and S. Yusuf (1999) Increased winter mortality from acute myocardial infarction and stroke: the effect of age. Journal of the American College of Cardiology 33(7):1916-1919.

Shimizu, M., Y. Hatta, H. Hayashi, M. Itokawa, Y. Yanagisawa, T. Otani, and N. Nakachi (1970) Effect of ascorbic acid on fibrinolysis. Acta Haemotologica Japonica 33(1):137-148.

Siegman, A., L. Kubzansky, I. Kawachi, S. Boyle, P. Vokonas, and D. Sparrow (2000) A prospective study of dominance and coronary artery disease in the Normative Aging Study. The American Journal of Cardiology 86(2):145-149.

Siegman, A., S. Townsend, A. Civelek, and R. Blumenthal (2000a) Antagonistic behavior, dominance, hostility, and coronary heart disease. Psychosomatic Medicine 62(2):248-257.

Simon, J. (1992) Vitamin C and cardiovascular disease: a review. Journal of the American College of Nutrition 11(2):107-125.

Simon, J., M. Murtaugh, M. Gross, C. Loria, S. Hulley, and D. Jacobs, Jr. (2004) Relation of ascorbic acid to coronary artery calcium. The Coronary Artery Risk Development in Young Adults Study. American Journal of Epidemiology 159(6):581-588.

Simpson, P. and B. Lucchesi (1987) Free radicals and myocardial ischemia and reperfusion injury. The Journal of Laboratory and Clinical Medicine 110(1):13-30.

Singh, D. and W. Chan (1974) Cardiomegaly and generalized oedema due to vitamin C deficiency. Singapore Medical Journal 15(1):60-63.

Singh, M., R. Singh, A. Khare, M. Gupta, N. Patney, V. Jain, S. Goyal, V. Prakash, and D. Pandey (1985) Serum copper in myocardial infarction—diagnostic and prognostic significance. Angiology 36(8):504-510.

Singh, R., M. Niaz, S. S. Rastogi, and S. Rastogi (1996) Usefulness of antioxidant vitamins in suspected acute myocardial infarction (the Indian experiment of infarct survival-3). The American Journal of Cardiology 77(4): 232-236.

Singhal, A. (2005) Endothelial dysfunction: role in obesity-related disorders and the early origins of CVD. The Proceedings of the Nutrition Society 64(1):15-22.

Sitaramayya, C. and T. Ali (1962) Studies on experimental hypercholesterolemia and atherosclerosis. Journal of Physiology and Pharmacology 6:192-204.

Smith, J., B. Niven, and J. Mann (1996) The effect of reduced extrinsic sucrose intake on plasma triglyceride levels. European Journal of Clinical Nutrition 50(8):498-504.

Soder, P., B. Soder, J. Nowak, and T. Jogestrand (2005) Early carotid atherosclerosis in subjects with periodontal diseases. Stroke: A Journal of Cerebral Circulation 36(6):1195-1200.

Sokoloff, B., M. Hori, C. Saelhof, T. Wrzolek, and T.
    Imai (1966) Aging, atherosclerosis and ascorbic acid
    metabolism. Journal of the American Geriatrics Society
    14(12):1239-1260.

Solajic-Bozicevic, N., A. Stavljenic, and M. Sesto (1991)
    Lecithin:cholesterol acyltransferase activity in patients
    with acute myocardial infarction and coronary heart
    disease. Artery 18(6):326-340.

Solajic-Bozicevic, N., A. Stavljenic-Rukavina, and M. Sesto
    (1994) Lecithin-cholesterol acyltransferase activity in
    patients with coronary artery disease examined by
    coronary angiography. The Clinical Investigator 72(12):
    951-956.

Solomon, H., R. Priore, and I. Bross (1968) Cigarette
    smoking and periodontal disease. Journal of the
    American Dental Association 77(5):1081-1084.

Som, S., S. Basu, D. Mukherjee, S. Deb, P. Choudhury,
    S. Mukherjee, S. Chatterjee, and I. Chatterjee (1981)
    Ascorbic acid metabolism in diabetes mellitus.
    Metabolism: Clinical and Experimental 30(6):572-577.

Sotres, L., G. van Huysen, and H. Gilmore (1969) A
    histologic study of gingival tissue response to
    amalgam, silicate and resin restorations. Journal of
    Periodontology 40(9):543-546.

Spencer, F., R. Goldberg, R. Becker, and J. Gore (1998)
    Seasonal distribution of acute myocardial infarction in
    the second National Registry of Myocardial Infarction.
    Journal of the American College of Cardiology 31(6):
    1226-1233.

Spittle, C., (1971) Atherosclerosis and vitamin C. The
    Lancet 2(7737):1280-1281.

Spittle, C. (1973) Vitamin C and deep-vein thrombosis.
    Lancet 2(7822):199-201.

Spittle, C. (1974) The action of vitamin C on blood vessels.
    American Heart Journal 88(3):387-388.

Stamler, J., R. Stamler, and K. Liu (1985) High blood pressure. In: Connor, W. and J. Bristow. (eds.) Coronary Heart Disease: Prevention, Complications, and Treatment. Philadelphia, PA: J.P. Lippincott Company.

Stankova, L., M. Riddle, J. Larned, K. Burry, D. Menashe, J. Hart, and R. Bigley (1984) Plasma ascorbate concentrations and blood cell dehydroascorbate transport in patients with diabetes mellitus. Metabolism: Clinical and Experimental 33(4):347-353.

Starkebaum, G. and J. Harlan (1986) Endothelial cell injury due to copper-catalyzed hydrogen peroxide generation from homocysteine. The Journal of Clinical Investigation 77(4):1370-1376.

Steinberg, D., S. Parthasarathy, T. Carew, J. Khoo, and J. Witztum (1989) Beyond cholesterol. Modifications of low-density lipoprotein that increase its atherogenicity. The New England Journal of Medicine 321(17):1196-1197.

Stemmermann, G., A. Nomura, L. Heilbrun, E. Pollack, and A. Kagan (1981) Serum cholesterol and colon cancer incidence in Hawaiian Japanese men. Journal of the National Cancer Institute 67(6):1179-1182.

Stevens, R., M. Colombo, J. Gonzales, W. Hollander, and K. Schmid (1976) The glycosaminoglycans of the human artery and their changes in atherosclerosis. The Journal of Clinical Investigation 58(2):470-481.

Steward, H., M. Bethea, S. Andrews, and L. Balart (1975) Sugar Busters! Cut Sugar to Trim Fat. New York, NY: Ballantine Books.

Stolman, J., H. Goldman, and B. Gould (1961) Ascorbic acid and blood vessels. Archives of Pathology 72:535-545.

Stone, I. (1976) Smoker's scurvy: orthomolecular preventive medicine in cigarette smoking. Orthomolecular Psychiatry 5(1):35-42.

Story, J. (1982) Dietary carbohydrate and atherosclerosis. Federation Proceedings 41(11):2797-2800.

Strauss, I. and P. Scheer (1939) Effect of nicotine on vitamin C metabolism. Internationale Zeitschrift fur Vitaminforschung 9:39-49.

Strauss, R. (2001) Environmental tobacco smoke and serum vitamin C levels in children. Pediatrics 107(3):540-542.

Stubbs, P., M. Seed, D. Moseley, B. O'Connor, P. Collinson, and M. Noble (1997) A prospective study of the role of lipoprotein(a) in the pathogenesis of unstable angina. European Heart Journal 18(4):603-607.

Subramanian, N., B. Nandi, A. Majumder, and I. Chatterjee (1973) Role of L-ascorbic acid on detoxification of histamine. Biochemical Pharmacology 22(13):1671-1673.

Sun, H., T. Koike, T. Ichikawa, K. Hatakeyama, M. Shiomi, B. Zhang, S. Kitajima, M. Morimoto, T. Watanabe, Y. Asada, Y. Chen, and J. Fan (2005) C-reactive protein in atherosclerotic lesions: its origin and pathophysiological significance. The American Journal of Pathology 167(4):1139-1148.

Szoke, von K., T. Zempleni, and L. Kallai (1963) Die wirkung gesteigerter kupferzufuhr auf den vitamin-C-haushalt von meerschweinchen bei parenteral zugefuhrter ascorbinsaure. Internationale Zeitschrift fur Vitaminforschung 33:175.

Tardif, J., J. Gregoire, and P. L'Allier (2002) Prevention of restenosis with antioxidants: mechanisms and implications. American Journal of Cardiovascular Drugs: Drugs, Devices, and Other Interventions 2(5): 323-334.

Tardif, J., J. Gregoire, L. Schwartz, L. Title, L. Laramee, F. Reeves, J. Lesperance, M. Bourassa, P. L'Allier, M. Glass, J. Lambert, M. Guertin; Canadian Antioxidant Restenosis Trial (CART-1) Investigators (2003) Effects of AGI-1067 and probucol after percutaneous coronary interventions. Circulation 107(4):552-558.

Tarugi, P., S. Calandra, P. Borella, and G. Vivoli (1982) Heavy metals and experimental atherosclerosis. Effect of lead intoxication on rabbit plasma lipoproteins. Atherosclerosis 45(2):221-234.

Tatsukawa, M., Y. Sawayama, N. Maeda, K. Okada, N. Furusyo, S. Kashiwagi, and J. Hayashi (2004) Carotid atherosclerosis and cardiovascular risk factors: a comparison of residents of a rural area of Okinawa with residents of a typical suburban area of Fukuoka, Japan. Atherosclerosis 172(2):337-343.

Taylor, A., J. Bindeman, I. Feuerstein, F. Cao, M. Brazaitis, and P. O'Malley (2005) Coronary calcium independently predicts incident premature coronary heart disease over measured cardiovascular risk factors. Mean three-year outcomes in the Prospective Army Coronary Calcium (PACC) Project. Journal of the American College of Cardiology 46(5):807-814.

Taylor, C., L. Nelson-Cox, B. Hall-Taylor, and G. Cox (1957) Atherosclerosis in monkeys with moderate hypercholesterolemia induced by dietary cholesterol. Federation Proceedings 16:374.

Taylor, C., G. Cox, and R. Trueheart (1961) Reversibility of atherosclerosis. Illinois Medical Journal 119:80-81.

Taylor, S. (1937) Scurvy and carditis. Lancet 1:973-979.

Teramoto, K., M. Daimon, R. Hasegawa, T. Toyoda, T. Sekine, T. Kawata, K. Yoshida, and I. Komuro (2005) Acute effect of oral vitamin C on coronary circulation in young healthy smokers. American Heart Journal 148(2):300-305.

Thubrikar, M. and F. Robicsek (1995) Pressure-induced arterial wall stress and atherosclerosis. The Annals of Thoracic Surgery 59(6):1594-1603.

Tillotson, J., G. Grandits, G. Bartsch, and J. Stamler (1997) Relation of dietary carbohydrates to blood lipids in the special intervention and usual care groups in the Multiple Risk Factor Intervention Trial. The American Journal of Clinical Nutrition 65(1 Suppl):314S-326S.

Tomoda, H., M. Yoshitake, K. Morimoto, and N. Aoki (1996) Possible prevention of postangioplasty restenosis by ascorbic acid. The American Journal of Cardiology 78(11):1284-1286.

Trieu, V., T. Zioncheck, R. Lawn, and W. McConathy (1991) Interaction of apolipoprotein(a) with apolipoprotein B-containing lipoproteins. Journal of Biological Chemistry 266(9):5480-5485.

Trivedi, S. and S. Talim (1973) The response of human gingival to restorative materials. The Journal of Prosthetic Dentistry 29(1):73-80.

Tunstall-Pedoe, H., M. Woodward, R. Tavendale, R. A'Brook, and M. McCluskey (1997) Comparison of the prediction by 27 different factors of coronary heart disease and death in men and women of the Scottish heart health study: cohort study. BMJ 315(7110):722-729.

Turgeon, J., L. LeMay, and R. Cleroux (1972) Periodontal effects of restoring proximal tooth surfaces with amalgam: a clinical evaluation in children. Journal of the Canadian Dental Association 38(7):255-256.

Turley, S., C. West, and B. Horton (1976) The role of ascorbic acid in the regulation of cholesterol metabolism and in the pathogenesis of atherosclerosis. Atherosclerosis 24(1-2):1-18.

Vaccarino, V., S. Kasl, J. Abramson, and H. Krumholz (2001) Depressive symptoms and risk of functional decline and death in patients with heart failure. Journal of the American College of Cardiology 38(1):199-205.

Valko, M., H. Morris, and M. Cronin (2005) Metals, toxicity and oxidative stress. Current Medicinal Chemistry 12(10):1161-1208.

Verlangieri, A. and R. Mumma (1973) In vivo sulfation of cholesterol by ascorbic acid 2-sulfate. Atherosclerosis 17(1):37-48.

Verlangieri, A. and J. Stevens (1979) L-ascorbic acid: effects on aortic glycosaminoglycan 35S incorporation in rabbit-induced atherogenesis. Blood Vessels 16(4):177-185.

Vita, J., J. Keaney, Jr., K. Raby, J. Morrow, J. Freedman, S. Lynch, S. Koulouris, B. Hankin, and B. Frei (1998) Low plasma ascorbic acid independently predicts the presence of an unstable coronary syndrome. Journal of the American College of Cardiology 31(5):980-986.

von Eckardstein, A., H. Schulte, P. Cullen, and G. Assmann (2001) Lipoprotein(a) further increases the risk of coronary events in men with high global cardiovascular risk. Journal of the American College of Cardiology 37(2):434-439.

Wall, R., J. Harlan, L. Harker, and G. Striker (1980) Homocysteine-induced endothelial cell injury in vitro: a model for the study of vascular injury. Thrombosis Research 18(1-2):113-121.

Wallberg, G. and G. Walldius (1982) Lack of effect of ascorbic acid on serum lipoprotein concentrations in patients with hypertriglyceridemia. Atherosclerosis 43(2-3):283-288.

Watson, K. and E. Kerr (1975) Functional role of cholesterol in infection and autoimmunity. Lancet 1(7902):308-310.

Weinhouse, S. and E. Hirsch (1940) Chemistry of atherosclerosis. I. Lipid and calcium content of the intima and of the media of the aorta with and without atherosclerosis. Archives of Pathology 29:31-41.

Weiss, S. (1989) Tissue destruction by neutrophils. The New England Journal of Medicine 320(6):365-376.

Wendt, M., C. Soparker, K. Louie, S. Basinger, and R. Gross (1997) Ascorbate stimulates type I and type III collagen in human Tenon's fibroblasts. Journal of Glaucoma 6(6):402-407.

Westhuyzen, J., A. Cochrane, P. Tesar, T. Mau, D. Cross, M. Frenneaux, F. Khafagi, and S. Fleming (1997) Effect of preoperative supplementation with alpha-tocopherol and ascorbic acid on myocardial injury in patients undergoing cardiac operations. The Journal of Thoracic and Cardiovascular Surgery 113(5):942-948.

Wick, G., M. Romen, A. Amberger, B. Metzler, M. Mayr, G. Falkensammer, and Q. Xu (1997) Atherosclerosis, autoimmunity, and vascular-associated lymphoid tissue. Federation of American Societies for Experimental Biology Journal 11(13):1199-1207.

Wiesel, J. (1906) Die erkrankungen arterieller gefasse im verlaufe acuter infectionen. Ztschr f Heilk, Wien u Leipz 27:262.

Wiesel, J. (1906a) Ueber erkrankungen der koronararterien im verlaufe acuter infektionskrankheiten. Wien Klin Wchnschr 19:723.

Wilens, S. (1947) The resorption of arterial atheromatous deposits in wasting disease. American Journal of Pathology 23:793-804.

Will, J. and T. Byers (1996) Does diabetes mellitus increase the requirement for vitamin C? Nutrition Reviews 54(7):193-202.

Will, J., E. Ford, and B. Bowman (1999) Serum vitamin C concentrations and diabetes: findings from the Third National Health and Nutrition Examination Survey, 1988-1994. American Journal of Clinical Nutrition 70(1): 49-52.

Williams, R., P. Sorlie, M. Feinleib, P. McNamara, W. Kannel, and T. Dawber (1981) Cancer incidence by levels of cholesterol. The Journal of the American Medical Association 245(3):247-252.

Willis, G. (1953) An experimental study of the intimal ground substance in atherosclerosis. Canadian Medical Association Journal 69:17-22.

Willis, G. (1957) The reversibility of atherosclerosis. Canadian Medical Association Journal 77:106-109.

Willis, G., A. Light, and W. Gow (1954) Serial arteriography in atherosclerosis. Canadian Medical Association Journal 71:562-568.

Willis, G. and S. Fishman (1955) Ascorbic acid content of human arterial tissue. Canadian Medical Association Journal 72:500-503.

Wilson, J. (2005) Regulation of vitamin C transport. Annual Review of Nutrition 25:105-125.

Wilson, T., S. Datta, J. Murrell, and C. Andrews (1973) Relation of vitamin C levels to mortality in a geriatric hospital: a study of the effect of vitamin C administration. Age and Ageing 2(3):163-171.

Wilson, T., C. Meservey, and R. Nicolosi (1998) Soy lecithin reduces plasma lipoprotein cholesterol and early atherogenesis in hypercholesterolemic monkeys and hamsters: beyond lineoleate. Atherosclerosis 140(1): 147-153.

Wolbach, S. and P. Howe (1926) Intercellular substances in experimental scorbutus. Archives of Pathology and Laboratory Medicine 1(1):1-24.

Wolff, S., Z. Jiang, and J. Hunt (1991) Protein glycation and oxidative stress in diabetes mellitus and ageing. Free Radical Biology & Medicine 10(5):339-352.

Xu, Q., S. Kiechl, M. Mayr, B. Metzler, G. Egger, F. Oberhollenzer, J. Willeit, and G. Wick (1999) Association of serum antibodies to heat-shock protein 65 with carotid atherosclerosis: clinical significance determined in a follow-up study. Circulation 100(11): 1169-1174.

Xu, Q., G. Schett, H. Perschinka, M. Mayr, G. Egger, F. Oberhollenzer, J. Willeit, S. Kiechl, and G. Wick (2000) Serum soluble heat shock protein 60 is elevated in subjects with atherosclerosis in a general population. Circulation 102(1):14-20.

Yang, F., H. Tan, and H. Wang (2005) Hyperhomocysteinemia and atherosclerosis. Sheng Li Xue Bao [Acta Physiologica Sinica] 57(2):103-114.

You, S. and Q. Wang (2005) Ferritin in atherosclerosis. Clinica Chimica Acta: International Journal of Clinical Chemistry 357(1):1-16.

Yousef, M., M. Salem, K. Kamel, G. Hassan, and F. El-Nouty (2003) Influence of ascorbic acid supplementation on the haematological and clinical biochemistry parameters of male rabbits exposed to aflatoxin B1. Journal of Environmental Science and Health. Part B. Pesticides, Food Contaminants, and Agricultural Wastes 38(2):193-209.

Yu, H. and N. Rifai (2000) High-sensitivity C-reactive protein and atherosclerosis: from theory to therapy. Clinical Biochemistry 33(8):601-610.

Yudkin, J. (1972) Sweet and Dangerous. New York, NY: Bantam Books, Inc.

Yudkin, J., O. Eisa, S. Kang, S. Meraji, and K. Bruckdorfer (1986) Dietary sucrose affects plasma HDL cholesterol concentration in young men. Annals of Nutrition & Metabolism 30(4):261-266.

Zaitsev, V., L. Myasnikov, L. Kasatkina, N. Lobova, and T. Sukasova (1964) The effect of ascorbic acid on experimental atherosclerosis. Cor et Vasa 6(1):19-25.

Zhang, J., X. Ying, Q. Lu, A. Kallner, R. Xiu, P. Henriksson, and I. Bjorkhem (1999) A single high dose of vitamin C counteracts the acute negative effect on microcirculation induced by smoking a cigarette. Microvascular Research 58(3):305-311.

Zheng, S., A. Ershow, C. Yang, G. Li, R. Li, H. Li, X. Zou. X. Liu, L. Song, Q. Qing, et al. (1989) Nutritional status in Linxian, China: effects of season and supplementation. International Journal for Vitamin and Nutrition Research 59(2):190-199.

Zieden, B. and A. Olsson (2005) The role of statins in the prevention of ischemic stroke. Current Atherosclerosis Reports 7(5):364-368.

Zyzanski, S., C. Jenkins, T. Ryan, A. Flessas, and M.
    Everist (1976) Psychological correlates of coronary
    angiographic findings. Archives of Internal Medicine
    136(11):1234-1237.